Progressive Tinnitus Management

Clinical Handbook for Audiologists

PTM

Progressive Tinnitus Management

Progressive Tinnitus Management

Clinical Handbook for Audiologists

James A. Henry
Tara L. Zaugg
Paula J. Myers
Caroline J. Kendall

Plural Publishing Inc.
San Diego
Oxford
Brisbane

PLURAL PUBLISHING INC.

5521 Ruffin Road
San Diego, CA 92123

e-mail: info@pluralpublishing.com
Web site: http://www.pluralpublishing.com

49 Bath Street
Abingdon, Oxfordshire OX14 1EA
United Kingdom

Typeset in 10½/13 Palatino by Flanagan's Publishing Services, Inc.
Printed in Canada by Transcontinental

Library of Congress Cataloging-in-Publication Data

Progressive tinnitus management : clinical handbook for audiologists / James A. Henry . . . [et al.].
p. ; cm.
Includes bibliographical references and index.
ISBN-13: 978-1-59756-404-5 (alk. paper)
ISBN-10: 1-59756-404-4 (alk. paper)
1. Tinnitus—Handbooks, manuals, etc. I. Henry, James, 1949-
[DNLM: 1. Tinnitus--rehabilitation. 2. Rehabilitation of Hearing Impaired--methods. WV 272 P964 2010]
RF293.8.P76 2010
617.8—dc22

2010004797

PTM

Progressive Tinnitus Management

Contents

Also Included:
DVD: "Managing Your Tinnitus" (for Level 3 group viewing)
CD: PowerPoint files (for Level 3 live presentations)

PTM

Progressive Tinnitus Management

Foreword

Tinnitus can dramatically compromise quality of life, rendering some persons unable to function as happy, healthy, and productive human beings. Tinnitus is one of the most common health concerns among combat-injured military personnel and veterans, and a major health care problem within the VA system. Tinnitus is also a significant health issue in the general population. Each year debilitating tinnitus prompts millions of persons to seek help from health care providers. Unfortunately, the person with tinnitus often does not benefit from prompt and appropriate care from physicians and other health care providers. Although effective tinnitus management techniques do exist, and all persons with bothersome tinnitus can be helped, a systematic, logical, and efficient approach to this large-scale health care problem is desperately needed. The progressive tinnitus management (PTM) method described in the new three-book Plural bundle offers such a solution.

The information within the three PTM books is evidence-based and clinically-proven. The strategy for assessment and management of tinnitus contained within the three books is consistent with the accumulated clinical experiences of audiologists who provide services to persons with bothersome tinnitus. In the words of the authors, PTM "utilizes a hierarchical structure for providing clinical services. That is, patients receive services that 'progress' to higher levels only as needed." For many (perhaps most) prospective patients, timely and accurate information about tinnitus coupled with rather generic counseling will allay their concerns and prevent the need for more extensive (and expensive) intervention. At the other end of the tinnitus seriousness spectrum are patients with disabling tinnitus and, often, complex health and audiologic histories including significant management challenges such as posttraumatic stress disorder (PTSD). This relatively small proportion of patients will require highly specialized and individualized support and management.

The authors of the three books—three audiologists and one psychologist—draw on years of research and clinical experience with tinnitus assessment and management in the development of the PTM approach. Readers are probably already familiar with the authors' peer-reviewed publications on tinnitus. James Henry, PhD is a VA Research Career Scientist at the National Center for Rehabilitative Auditory Research (NCRAR). Tara Zaugg, AuD is a research audiologist at the NCRAR. Paula Myers, PhD is Chief of the Audiology Section and Cochlear Implant Coordinator at the James A. Haley VA Hospital in Tampa, Florida. Caroline Kendall, PhD is a research psychologist at the VA Connecticut Healthcare System in West Haven Connecticut.

Multiple unique features of the three PTM books contribute importantly to their clinical usefulness. The first book of the bundle is a clinical handbook on PTM written for audiologists. The components of the progressive tinnitus management approach are thoroughly explained in nine chapters. Clinical implementation of PTM is facilitated with 25 appendices containing a variety of practical materials such as patient handouts, questionnaires, and procedural guides. The handbook also includes a clinically valuable CD with informational PowerPoint presentations plus a DVD containing videos for patients containing, for example, demonstrations of different relaxation techniques. The second book is a guide for one-on-one counseling of patients with tinnitus. In the management of bothersome tinnitus and hyperacusis (reduced sound tolerance), patient counseling is an essential and very effective component of intervention. The 300-page counseling guidebook is designed and formatted to be used directly in the counseling process, literally interfacing the audiologist with the patient. The counseling book also includes a 75-minute audio CD with a variety of sound tracks to demonstrate different types of sounds that can be used for managing reactions to tinnitus.

Consistent with the clinically proven adage that "knowledge is power," the third book is a self-help workbook written for the person with tinnitus. The workbook provides step-by-step instructions to facilitate learning how to self-manage reactions to tinnitus. It also includes information on hearing protection, relaxation exercises, cognitive behavioral therapy (CBT) and 10 appendices chock full of additional practical information prepared for the patient. The self-help workbook will be very useful to augment the services provided by audiologists, and also will be invaluable for patients who, for various reasons, cannot directly access the services of an audiologist.

The three PTM books, with varied accompanying educational materials, provide a remarkably creative and comprehensive solution for the health care problem of tinnitus in both the VA and non-VA patient populations. Most audiologists regularly encounter patients who require a compassionate and evidence-based approach for diagnosis and intervention for bothersome tinnitus. Within the PTM book series is all the information and materials an audiologist needs to provide effective clinical services to this traditionally underserved patient population.

James W. Hall III, PhD
University of Florida

PTM

Progressive Tinnitus Management

Introduction

Tinnitus is the perception of sound in the ears or head that does not have a source outside the body. The perceived sound is generated within the body and thus has been referred to as a "phantom" sound. Most typically, people who experience tinnitus have been exposed to loud noise that caused damage to the auditory system, resulting in both tinnitus and hearing loss. There are numerous other causes of tinnitus, as reviewed in Chapter 1.

Tinnitus is a vexing and intractable problem for millions of people. It can cause sleep problems, difficulty concentrating, and can be the cause of mental health problems—most commonly anxiety and depression. People who already suffer from mental health conditions may be particularly vulnerable to tinnitus becoming problematic. Interestingly, of all the people who experience tinnitus, many more are *not* bothered by it than those who are. This is just one of many aspects of tinnitus that make it difficult to provide a clinical program that addresses the needs of all patients who report tinnitus to a health care provider.

We have conducted tinnitus clinical research at the Portland VA Medical Center continuously since 1995 (under the auspices of the VA National Center for Rehabilitative Auditory Research since 1997). Our initial studies evaluated psychoacoustic aspects of tinnitus. In 1999 we started the first of a series of controlled clinical studies to evaluate different methods of tinnitus intervention (as described in Chapter 2). These clinical studies provided important efficacy data with respect to the different methods studied, but more importantly we learned a great deal about how best to meet the needs of patients who suffer from tinnitus.

We determined that a "progressive" approach to tinnitus management was essential to most efficiently address the range of services needed by patients. In 2006 we received a research grant from VA Rehabilitation, Research and Development (RR&D) Service to develop and test a new method that was progressive in its approach. The method was designed to be conducted entirely by audiologists, provided patients were referred appropriately to other disciplines as needed. Five hierarchical levels of clinical services were defined, and patients "progressed" only to the level of care necessary to meet their needs. The intervention mainly was educational and was intended to promote self-efficacy for managing reactions to tinnitus. The overall intent was to meet the needs of patients on an individualized basis, and to provide them with the self-management skills that they would likely need for a lifetime.

Following development of our progressive approach, it became clear that psychological effects due to tinnitus needed to be addressed. This resulted in the incorporation of cognitive-behavioral therapy (CBT) into the intervention protocol. CBT has been used for many years as effective intervention for pain, depression, and anxiety. CBT was adapted to the management of tinnitus and was shown to be effective with many people for that purpose. We now have incorporated key components of CBT into the PTM program, resulting in an interdisciplinary approach to providing tinnitus clinical services.

The result of these efforts is the development of progressive tinnitus management (PTM). The method continues to evolve, especially with the addition of CBT. However, the method has reached a level of development at which it now can be specifically defined with respect to the procedures required for its clinical implementation. This book provides a description of the clinical procedures necessary for audiologists to conduct PTM. A separate book is in preparation that will focus primarily on CBT procedures used by mental health specialists to combine with the audiologic components of PTM.

It is acknowledged that numerous methods of tinnitus management are in use and that clinicians often disagree regarding the most effective approach. A number of controlled clinical studies have been completed that demonstrate benefit to the majority of participants enrolled in these studies. However, these studies are not definitive; thus, clinicians have the latitude to use any method that has research support. It is important to recognize that evidence-based tinnitus interventions use some combination of three broad components: education, relaxation techniques, and therapeutic sound. Addressing some or all of these three components in general provides reasonable benefit such that many patients notice a significant improvement in their quality of life. Of course, there is no cure for tinnitus; thus, patients must realize that no matter which method is applied, their tinnitus perception will most likely remain unchanged and that clinical management focuses on reducing any negative reactions associated with the tinnitus.

Although many practitioners already are conducting some form of tinnitus therapy, others have little to no experience providing tinnitus services. Experienced clinicians generally have definite ideas about how to go about providing tinnitus services to their patients. These clinicians can adopt PTM as described in this book, or they can use the different levels of PTM as a framework within which to conduct their preferred form of therapy. For clinicians with little to no experience, it is suggested they start by implementing the first three levels of PTM. With sufficient experience implementing these lower levels, they can start practicing the higher levels (Levels 4 and 5).

The interdisciplinary aspect of PTM requires some further explanation. Level 1 Triage is directed to all clinicians (except audiologists or other ear specialists) who encounter patients complaining of bothersome tinnitus. Nonaudiologist clinicians are provided with guidelines to assist them in properly referring these patients for appropriate clinical services. Level 2 Audiologic Evaluation is performed solely by audiologists who: (a) conduct an auditory assessment; (b) facilitate management of any hearing disorders; (c) conduct a brief assessment of tinnitus impact; and (d) (optional) provide educational materials to the patient to facilitate self-management. Level 3 Group Education involves two interactive workshops conducted by an audiologist, which focus on teaching patients how to use therapeutic sound. In addition, a psychologist (or other qualified mental health professional) conducts three workshops that teach key principles of CBT. The CBT sessions are designed to facilitate specific coping skills to augment the use of therapeutic sound.

Although it is optimal that a mental health provider be part of the PTM clinical team, we recognize that this will not always be possible. At a minimum, appropriate mental health providers should be identified and then used to refer patients when mental health services are needed. Audiologists should take the lead in implementing PTM, and adapt the program as necessary to be flexible in how it is implemented to make the most of the resources available at any one clinic.

Patients whose needs are not met through Level 3 are advised to undergo Level 4 Interdisciplinary Evaluation. The evaluation should be conducted by both an audiologist and a mental health professional (typically a psychologist, as they are specifically trained to evaluate and diagnose mental health disorders). The audiologist and psychologist work as a team for Levels 4 and 5 collaboratively to determine the best therapeutic approach for the patient. Level 5 Individualized Support thus can involve multiple appointments with the audiologist, the psychologist, or both. Level 5 normally involves up to 6 months of individualized support. Throughout each level, the goal of intervention is for the patient to learn the skills necessary to self-manage any situation in which his or her tinnitus is problematic.

This handbook provides minimal background information about tinnitus and focuses on describing the practical information that is necessary to learn how to implement PTM in the clinic. Chapter 1 establishes common ground with respect to terminology and definitions pertaining to tinnitus management. Chapter 2 describes how our controlled clinical studies (and other influences) led to the development of PTM. Chapter 3 provides an overview of PTM. The remaining chapters detail the clinical procedures that are used for each of the five levels of PTM. These details include numerous forms, questionnaires, clinical "cheat-sheets," and patient handouts—all of which are provided as appendices.

The goal of intervention with PTM is for patients to learn how to develop and implement individualized plans to manage their reactions to tinnitus. These plans involve the use of therapeutic sound and coping techniques. Success in achieving this goal depends largely on patients acquiring confidence in applying the self-management strategies. Breaking the process of learning into small achievable tasks helps to ensure that patients experience initial success. This approach is consistent with the self-efficacy theory. Research has demonstrated that self-efficacy is a good predictor of motivation and behavior. In general, the experience of success increases self-efficacy whereas experiencing failure reduces self-efficacy. This is a basic tenet of intervention with PTM.

Clinical implementation of PTM by audiologists should involve the use of two additional books that were prepared to facilitate educating patients in the self-management techniques. The first is a self-help workbook (*How to Manage Your Tinnitus: A Step-by-Step Guide*) for patients that provides step-by-step procedures to learn how to develop individualized plans for managing their reactions to tinnitus—one using therapeutic sound and the other using selected coping techniques from CBT. The workbook includes videos that model much of what is taught during Level 3 Group Education, as well as a CD that describes and demonstrates the various uses of therapeutic sound.

The second book (*Progressive Tinnitus Management: Counseling Guide*) is a patient counseling guide that is used by audiologists during Level 5 Individualized Support. The book lays flat between the clinician and patient, and is used like a flip chart—each time a page is turned, the page facing the clinician provides talking points while the opposite page faces the patient and provides short bullet points plus graphics that illustrate the main points. A second counseling guide is being developed for psychologists to implement the CBT components of PTM during Level 5.

PTM has been developed to a high degree of specificity, but it is important to realize that the methodology is considered a "work in progress." We are learning continually, from both patients and clinicians, and the methodology is revised to be appropriately responsive to this feedback. Audiologists are encouraged to modify the materials and procedures as necessary to meet the needs of their patients and their clinics.

It is our sincere hope that this handbook will provide you with information that ultimately will result in improved outcomes for your patients who need help learning how to manage their reactions to tinnitus. We always welcome your comments and suggestions to continually improve on these methods.

PTM

Progressive Tinnitus Management

Acknowledgments

Development and publication of this book was supported by the VA Rehabilitation Research and Development (RR&D) Service, the NCRAR, and VA Employee Education System. Numerous individuals have contributed in various and significant ways toward this effort, including:

- **Daniel C. Garcia** (Graphic Designer, Long Beach Employee Education Resource Center, Long Beach, California)
- **Katie J. Fick, MS** (Research Assistant, James A. Haley Veterans' Hospital, Tampa, Florida)
- **Christine Kaelin, MBA** (Clinical Research Coordinator, NCRAR, Portland, Oregon)
- **Robert Kerns, PhD** (National Program Director for Pain Management, Veterans Health Administration, VA Connecticut Healthcare System, West Haven, Connecticut)
- **David Lehman** (Executive Producer, Salt Lake City Employee Education Resource Center, Salt Lake City, Utah)
- **Marcia Legro, PhD** (Research Psychologist, Seattle, Washington)
- **Will Murphy** (Audiovisual Production Specialist, Portland VA Medical Center)
- **Kimberly Owens, MPH** (Clinical Research Coordinator, Saint Thomas Research Institute, Nashville, Tennessee)
- **Martin Schechter, PhD** (Audiologist, Portland VA Medical Center)
- **Emily Thielman, MS** (Research Assistant, NCRAR, Portland, Oregon)
- **Dwayne Washington** (Audiovisual Production Specialist, Portland VA Medical Center)
- **John C. Whatley, PhD** (Project Manager, Birmingham Employee Education Resource Center, Birmingham, Alabama)

Also, thanks to Stephen Fausti, PhD and Sara Ruth Oliver, AuD for their continued support of tinnitus research and clinical activities at the Portland VA Medical Center. Illustrations were done by Lynn Kitagawa, MFA, Medical Media Service, VA Medical Center, Portland, Oregon.

Authors and Contributors

James A. Henry, PhD
VA RR&D National Center for Rehabilitative Auditory Research (NCRAR) at the Portland VA Medical Center,
Portland, Oregon;
and Department of Otolaryngology,
Oregon Health and Science University,
Portland, Oregon

Caroline J. Kendall, PhD
VA Connecticut Healthcare System,
West Haven, Connecticut;
and Department of Psychiatry, Yale University,
New Haven, Connecticut

Paula J. Myers, PhD
VA Audiology Clinic, James A. Haley Veterans' Hospital,
Tampa, Florida

Tara L. Zaugg, AuD
VA RR&D National Center for Rehabilitative Auditory Research at the Portland VA Medical Center,
Portland, Oregon

Special Contributions by:

Marcia Legro, PhD (Chapter 2)

Kyle Dennis, PhD (Chapter 3)

Dennis Trune, PhD (Chapter 4)

Elias Michaelides, MD (Chapter 5)

Kathryn Sanders, PhD (Chapter 5)

Lynn Kitagawa, MFA (Illustrations)

This book is dedicated to our nation's military veterans. We thank you for serving our country. You are the reason we enjoy freedom.

1

Definitions and Background

PTM

Progressive Tinnitus Management

Tinnitus is a surprisingly complex subject. Numerous books would be required to adequately cover the current body of knowledge. The present handbook focuses on describing procedures for providing clinical services for tinnitus using the methodology of progressive tinnitus management (PTM).

In this opening chapter we establish common ground with respect to terminology and contextual information. Relevant definitions are provided, many of which are operational due to lack of consensus in the field. Additional background information includes brief descriptions of epidemiologic data, patient data, and conditions related to reduced tolerance (hypersensitivity) to sound.

Basic Concepts and Terminology

Tinnitus is the experience of perceiving sound that is not produced by a source outside of the body. The "phantom" auditory perception is generated somewhere in the auditory pathways or in the head or neck. Tinnitus often is referred to as "ringing in the ears." And, in fact, the word "tinnitus" is derived from the Latin word *tinniere*, which means "to ring." Patients report many different sounds—not just ringing—when describing the sound of their tinnitus, as we discuss later in this chapter.

Transient Ear Noise

It seems that almost everyone experiences "transient ear noise," which typically is described as a sudden whistling sound accompanied by the perception of hearing loss (Kiang, Moxon, & Levine, 1970). No systematic studies have been published to date describing the prevalence and properties of transient ear noise; thus, anything known about this phenomenon is anecdotal.

The transient auditory event is unilateral and seems to occur completely at random without anything precipitating the sudden onset of symptoms. Often the ear feels blocked during the episode. The symptoms generally dissipate within a period of about a minute. Although transient ear noise has been described as "brief spontaneous tinnitus"

(Dobie, 2004b), any reference to tinnitus in this book does not include this auditory phenomenon.

Chronic Tinnitus

Patients often confuse transient ear noise with chronic tinnitus. What differentiates the two? It has been suggested that tinnitus is ear noise that lasts at least five minutes (Coles, 1984; A. C. Davis, 1995; Hazell, 1995). Dauman and Tyler (1992) suggested that the noise must last at least five minutes *and* occur at least two times per week. These are reasonable criteria to define tinnitus, but superfluous for the typical patient who experiences tinnitus all or most of the time. Nonetheless, a distinction must be made between transient ear noise and chronic tinnitus, and Dauman and Tyler's criteria are sufficient for this purpose.

Origin of Tinnitus: Somatic Versus Neurophysiologic

By definition, the *perception* of tinnitus results from activity in the auditory nervous system. The neural activity that is perceived as tinnitus can be referred to as a "tinnitus neural signal." As for most sounds that activate the auditory system, at any point in time the tinnitus neural signal may or may not be part of the conscious experience. Whenever tinnitus is consciously perceived, the tinnitus neural signal is undergoing active processing by the auditory cortex (J. A. Henry, Trune, Robb, & Jastreboff, 2007a). Although the final destination of the tinnitus neural signal always is the auditory cortex, the *origin* of tinnitus can be from either outside or within the auditory nervous system (referred to as *somatic* and *neurophysiologic* tinnitus, respectively) (Hazell, 1998a).

If the tinnitus has a somatic origin, it can be referred to as *somatic tinnitus* or *somatosound(s)*. If the tinnitus has a neurophysiologic origin, it can be referred to as *neurophysiologic tinnitus* or *sensorineural tinnitus*. The word *tinnitus* generally refers to neurophysiologic tinnitus because this is the condition that is experienced by the great majority of patients.

Somatic Tinnitus (Somatosound)

Somatic tinnitus *(somatosound)* has an origin that usually is vascular, muscular, skeletal, respiratory, or located in the temporomandibular joint (TMJ) (J. A. Henry, Dennis, & Schechter, 2005). These "body sounds" thus have an internal acoustic source (Dobie, 2004b). Theoretically, the acoustic signal associated with any somatosound could be detected and characterized if the proper sensing equipment were available for this purpose.

Somatosound—Pulsatile Tinnitus

The most common type of somatosound is *pulsatile* tinnitus (Lockwood, Burkard, & Salvi, 2004). Also referred to as *venous hum* or *vascular noise*, pulsatile tinnitus pulses in synchrony with the heartbeat (Sismanis, 2003). There are many potential sites for pulsatile tinnitus, which often can be identified by an experienced physician (Lockwood et al., 2004; Sismanis, 1998; Wackym & Friedland, 2004). It is essential that these patients receive a medical examination as pulsatile tinnitus might indicate a more serious medical problem (such as intracranial and carotid artery abnormalities) (Hazell, 1990; Sismanis, 2007). The condition is treatable in some patients (Sismanis, 1998).

Nonpulsatile Somatosounds

Somatosounds also can be *nonpulsatile*, meaning that they have a nonvascular source (typically muscular, respiratory, or TMJ). Examples of nonvascular conditions that can cause somatosounds are muscular flutters or spasms and patulous eustachian tube.

Symptoms of Somatosounds

When evaluating a patient who complains of tinnitus, it is essential to determine if the symptoms suggest a somatic origin. If so, then the possibility exists that the tinnitus is amenable to medical management. Information about diagnosing somatic tinnitus is available in several publications (Hazell, 1990; Levine, 2004; Perry & Gantz, 2000; Schwaber, 2003; Wackym & Friedland, 2004). (Please see Chapters 4 and 5 for further information about somatosounds.)

Somatosounds Require Medical Evaluation

The presence of somatosounds always indicates the need for medical evaluation. The physician (usually an otolaryngologist or otologist) should have expertise in the diagnosis and treatment of somatic tinnitus. If the physician cannot resolve the problem with medical or surgical intervention, then the audiologist should provide appropriate clinical services, as described in later chapters.

Neurophysiologic (Sensorineural) Tinnitus

By far the majority of patients who complain of tinnitus have *neurophysiologic* (or *sensorineural*) tinnitus, that is, tinnitus that originates somewhere within the auditory nervous system. Although there is no known cure for neurophysiologic tinnitus, patients can learn to manage their reactions to tinnitus, thereby improving quality of life.

Origin of Neurophysiologic Tinnitus

All we can know for certain about the origin of a patient's sensorineural tinnitus is that it is generated somewhere within the auditory nervous system. The cochlea seems a likely site because damage to the cochlea from noise exposure and other factors often results in tinnitus. However, some desperate patients have undergone surgical severing of cranial nerve VIII, which extends from the cochlea to the brain, although it did not stop their tinnitus (Fisch, 1970; House & Brackmann, 1981; Pulec, 1984). This finding indicated that tinnitus can be generated centrally. Evidence is accumulating that supports the central generation of tinnitus (Møller, 2003). Cacace (2003) proposed that central networks of auditory system neurons may be involved in generating and sustaining tinnitus, which would explain the persistence of tinnitus following auditory nerve transection.

Understanding the pathophysiology of sensorineural tinnitus is a goal that is being pursued by an ever increasing number of researchers. Many theories have been proposed regarding tinnitus etiology, but are beyond the scope of this clinically oriented book. The interested reader has a choice of myriad publications written on this topic (e.g., Bauer, 2004; Eggermont & Roberts, 2004; P. J. Jastreboff, 1990; Kaltenbach, Zhang, & Finlayson, 2005; Kaltenbach, Zhang, & Zacharek, 2004; Nuttall, Meikle, & Trune, 2004; Vernon & Møller, 1995).

Neurophysiologic Tinnitus Is a Phantom Auditory Perception

Phantom sensations such as phantom pain and phantom limb have characteristics that are analogous to those of tinnitus (P. J. Jastreboff, 1990, 1995; Meikle, 1995; Møller, 2003). Tinnitus thus has been referred to as a *phantom auditory perception* (P. J. Jastreboff, 1990). Pain and tinnitus are similar with respect to their physiology, assessment, and treatment (Møller, 1987, 2000). These analogous conditions also may have similar neuropathic generating mechanisms. Because of these similarities, strategies of pain management can offer valuable clues to the management of tinnitus. In fact, the method of psychotherapy, cognitive-behavioral therapy (CBT), has been shown to be effective in treating chronic pain (P. H. Wilson, J. L. Henry, & Nicholas, 1993). The success of CBT for the treatment of pain led to the development of CBT for tinnitus (J. L. Henry & P. H. Wilson, 2001).

Subjective Versus Objective Tinnitus

Objective Tinnitus

By definition, *objective tinnitus* is tinnitus that is audible to the examiner (Dobie, 2004b). Objective tinnitus is relatively rare and always is a somatosound with an internal acoustic source (which as already discussed indicates an underlying condition requiring a medical evaluation by an otolaryngologist or otologist). Not all somatosounds are detectable by the examiner, and thus not all somatosounds would meet the definition of objective tinnitus. As a somatosound is an acoustically generated signal, the signal should be detectable with proper measurement techniques.

Subjective Tinnitus

Subjective tinnitus is perceived only by the patient. Any description of subjective tinnitus comes only from the patient, as there are no means to directly measure the intensity or other characteristics of the tinnitus. *Tinnitus matching* is performed to *indirectly* measure subjective tinnitus, (J. A. Henry, 2004; J. A. Henry, Zaugg, & Schechter, 2005a). For the remainder of this book, the word *tinnitus* generally refers to subjective tinnitus, that is, to neurophysiologic or sensorineural tinnitus that does not have an internal acoustic source. When patients have somatosounds, behavioral methods can be applied to manage reactions to these sounds if medical management does not resolve the symptoms.

Auditory Imagery, Auditory Hallucinations, and Musical Hallucinations

Auditory imagery, auditory hallucinations, and musical hallucinations are different forms of phantom auditory perceptions. There often is confusion about how these different auditory perceptions differ from tinnitus.

Auditory Imagery

Auditory imagery is a normal phenomenon that occurs for all people. It generally refers to the *imagination of sound*, such as repeating a phone number in one's head, or recalling a musical passage (Kraemer, Macrae, Green, & Kelley, 2005; Seal, Aleman, & McGuire, 2004). "Auditory imaginations" can be under conscious control, but they also can occur outside of conscious control. When not under conscious control, auditory imaginations can be mildly distressing, as when you have a song "stuck in your head."

Auditory Hallucinations

Auditory hallucinations have been estimated to occur in 10 to 15% of the general population (Nicolson, Mayberg, Pennell, & Nemeroff, 2006; Sommer et al., 2008). Perhaps surprisingly, of those who experience auditory hallucinations, most do not have a psychotic disorder. In the nonpsychiatric population, auditory hallucinations have been described in conjunction with various diseases, injury, trauma, bereavement, sensory deprivation, religious experiences, near-death experiences, and drugs (Nicolson et al., 2006). Auditory hallucinations also may have nothing to do with the ability to hear, as people born profoundly deaf can experience them (du Feu & McKenna, 1999; Schonauer, Achtergarde, Gotthardt, & Folkerts, 1998).

Auditory hallucinations occur in 70 to 80% of patients with schizophrenia (Hugdahl et al., 2008). Auditory hallucinations normally ascribed to psychiatric illness can be perceived as "voices, cries, noises, or rarely, music" (Wengel, Burke, & Holemon, 1989, p. 163). Musical hallucinations, however, are not necessarily associated with psychopathology, and tend to occur in people with advancing age and marked hearing loss (Sacks, 2008). Bauman (2004) has distinguished "two basic types of auditory hallucinations—psychiatric auditory hallucinations and nonpsychiatric auditory hallucinations. People with mental illnesses often experience the former, while people who are hard of hearing often experience the latter" (pp. 17–18). Focusing on the latter, nonpsychiatric, type, Bauman makes the following points:

- Auditory hallucinations can consist of music, sounds, or voices.
- "Unformed" auditory hallucinations sound distorted and indistinct, whereas "formed" auditory hallucinations sound clear and recognizable.
- Auditory hallucinations typically are experienced by hard of hearing, socially isolated, elderly people who also have tinnitus.
- People who experience auditory hallucinations typically don't admit to the experience.
- At least 10% of hard of hearing people experience auditory hallucinations.
- Many people actually find auditory hallucinations to be pleasant. Based on this information, it is reasonable to expect some patients to report auditory hallucinations that are not associated with psychopathology.

If a patient who reports auditory hallucinations remains unconvinced that the sounds do not have an external acoustic source, then the experience may indicate presence of comorbid mental illness. In addition, the psychiatric population tends to experience auditory hallucinations as frequent, intrusive, and distressing, whereas the nonpsychiatric population may experience them as more positive and nonthreatening (Choong, Hunter, & Woodruff, 2007). One study has reported data suggesting that auditory hallucinations that occur in nonpsychiatric individuals suggest a general susceptibility to schizophrenia (Sommer et al., 2008).

Whenever auditory hallucinations are reported, patients should be referred to both audiology and mental health for a thorough history and to evaluate the auditory experiences—to determine if the sounds are tinnitus or auditory hallucinations and to determine if mental illness is involved.

Permanent Versus Temporary Tinnitus

Tinnitus can be a temporary or a permanent condition.

Permanent Tinnitus

It is, of course, impossible to determine if and when a person's tinnitus becomes permanent. In general, the longer a person has experienced tinnitus the more likely it is to be permanent. A general guideline is that tinnitus of at least 12 months duration has a high likelihood of being a permanent condition (Dobie, 2004b). However, it also has been suggested that a person must have experienced tinnitus for at least two years before it should be considered permanent (Vernon, 1996).

Temporary Tinnitus

Exposure to loud noise can cause temporary threshold shift as well as temporary tinnitus (Nuttall et al., 2004). Tinnitus induced in this fashion likely will resolve within a few days following the insult. Repeated episodes of noise exposure increase the likelihood that the tinnitus will become permanent.

Tinnitus also can be induced by a number of medications and drug interactions (DiSorga, 2001) (see Chapter 5). Such tinnitus usually is temporary (typically lasting 1 to 2 weeks postexposure), but can be permanent—especially with the use of aminoglycoside antibiotics or the cancer chemotherapeutic drug cisplatin (Fausti, J. A. Henry, & Frey, 1995; Rachel, Kaltenbach, & Janisse, 2002). Aspirin (containing salicylate) is well known to cause temporary tinnitus, although the dosage generally has to be rather high to induce tinnitus (Eggermont, 2004; Puel & Guitton, 2007). Other medications that can cause temporary tinnitus include NSAIDS, loop diuretics, and quinine. Drugs used to treat mental health and sleep conditions also may trigger or exacerbate tinnitus. Patients have reported exacerbation of tinnitus due to alcohol and caffeine.

Onset of Tinnitus

The onset of tinnitus is described as *gradual* for some and *sudden* for others (Axelsson & Barrenas, 1992). In a population study of older adults with tinnitus, 55% reported a gradual onset, 24% reported a sudden onset, and 21% did not know (Sindhusake, Golding, et al., 2003). Uncertainty about the onset of tinnitus can make it difficult to identify a precipitating event. Indeed, as discussed further below, many patients are unable to identify anything that was associated with the onset of their tinnitus.

Recent-Onset Tinnitus

Some patients report that they have experienced tinnitus for only a short period of time, usually measured in weeks or up to a few months. For these patients with *recent-onset tinnitus*, it first is important to rule out vestibular schwannoma or any other medical condition that might be causing the symptoms (which is routine practice for audiologists). If medical causes can be ruled out, an attempt should be made to determine if psychological factors such as stress, anxiety, depression, or lifestyle changes might have triggered the tinnitus onset. Patients always should be questioned about any exposure to loud noise. Identifying a potentially triggering event helps to focus the counseling most appropriately.

Patients with recent-onset tinnitus are particularly susceptible to acquiring fears or concerns that the internal sound indicates the presence of a serious medical condition. These patients may be quite anxious about the potential ramifications of the auditory symptoms. It therefore is critical to provide them with only positive and reassuring information to allay any fears. They should be counseled that (a) their tinnitus may be a temporary condition; (b) they should protect their ears in the presence of damaging sound (or to avoid loud sounds entirely) to optimize the potential for spontaneous resolution of the tinnitus; (c) tinnitus often raises concerns when it is new, but most people who have long-term tinnitus are not particularly bothered by it (Dobie, 2004b; Hallam, Rachman, & Hinchcliffe, 1984); and (d) if the tinnitus becomes bothersome to feel welcome to contact or return to the clinic to discuss ways to manage their reactions to it.

Some patients may remain unconvinced that the recent-onset tinnitus does not indicate a more serious condition, even after thorough audiologic and medical evaluations. These patients may need to be referred to a mental health clinician for assessment of comorbid psychological conditions.

Delayed-Onset Tinnitus

Delayed-onset tinnitus is thought to occur weeks, months, or even years following some precipitating event (e.g., exposure to loud noise, traumatic brain injury, treatment with ototoxic medications, etc.). It is not uncommon for patients to make a claim of delayed-onset tinnitus for litigation purposes. The possibility of such a claim being valid relates to the complex interaction among the presumed precursor event and more recent events that might have triggered the tinnitus onset. Evaluating a claim of delayed-onset tinnitus requires taking a detailed history that covers all possible circumstances that might have caused damage to the auditory system.

A better understanding of the mechanisms of tinnitus generation is needed before the existence of delayed onset of tinnitus can be positively confirmed or rejected (Humes, Joellenbeck, & Durch, 2006). However, it does seem likely that noise exposure or other experiences that could have caused auditory damage can result in delayed-onset tinnitus, even when the tinnitus onset occurs years after the event.

Epidemiology of Tinnitus

Prevalence of Tinnitus

Prevalence estimates from numerous epidemiologic studies indicate that about 10 to 15% of all adults experience tinnitus (H. J. Hoffman & Reed, 2004). The American Tinnitus Association (ATA) estimates that 40 to 50 million Americans experience tinnitus as a chronic condition and that of these, 10 to 12 million seek some form of medical help, and 2.5 million are "debilitated" by their tinnitus (S. C. Brown, 1990). Men have a higher incidence of tinnitus than women, likely due to occupational and recreational differences (H. J. Hoffman & Reed, 2004; Meikle & Walsh, 1984).

"Causes" of Tinnitus

We often refer to "causes" of tinnitus (i.e., tinnitus *etiology*), but in fact we never know the specific cause of sensorineural tinnitus (J. A. Henry, Dennis, et al., 2005). For example, we may say that noise exposure "caused" a person's tinnitus. The noise probably caused some cochlear damage, but it did not *cause* the tinnitus. Technically, instead of "causes," we should use terminology that implies indirect causality, such as *precipitating factors, events associated with tinnitus onset, tinnitus precursor events,* and *tinnitus triggering events.*

Auditory Pathologies Associated with Tinnitus

Numerous auditory pathologies have been associated with tinnitus. Sweetow (1996) has listed these with respect to conductive and sensorineural auditory pathologies (Table 1–1). It is important to realize that anything that can cause hearing loss also can trigger the onset of tinnitus (Coles, 1995; Dobie, 2004b).

Risk Factors

A number of studies have obtained tinnitus epidemiology data in a systematic fashion. H. J. Hoffman and Reed (2004) reviewed these studies and summarized the various factors that were shown

Table 1–1. Auditory Pathologies Associated With Tinnitus

Conductive	*Sensorineural*
Impacted cerumen	Endolymphatic hydrops
External otitis	Perilymph fistulas
Tympanic membrane perforations	Noise damage
Otitis media	Vestibular schwannoma
External auditory meatus tumors	Presbycusis
Cholesteatoma	Viral diseases
Ossicular chain fixation or discontinuity	Bacterial infections
Atresias	Ototoxicity
Otosclerosis	Meningionoma
Carcinoma	And so forth
And so forth	

Source: Sweetow (1996).

Table 1–2. Risk Factors for Tinnitus

"Definite" Risk Factors	*"Possible" Risk Factors*
Acoustic neuroma	Alcohol
Age	Anxiety
Cardiovascular and cerebrovascular disease	Depression
Drugs or medications	Familial inheritance
Ear infections/inflammation	Geographic region
Head/neck trauma and injury	Health status—fair/poor
Hyper- and hypothyroidism	Heavy weight or high body mass index
Loud noise exposure	Limited education
Ménière's disease	Low height
Otosclerosis	Low socioeconomic status
Presbycusis	Low weight or low body mass index
Sudden deafness	Rural residence
	Smoking (cigarettes)

Source: Adapted from "Epidemiology of Tinnitus," by H. J. Hoffman & G. W. Reed, 2004, in *Tinnitus: Theory and Management* by J. B. Snow (Ed.), (pp. 16–41), Lewiston, NY: BC Decker Inc. Copyright 2004 BC Decker, Inc. Adapted with permission.

to be associated with tinnitus. Their summary is divided between "definite" and "possible" risk factors (Table 1–2). Thus, people are "definitely" or "possibly" more likely to have tinnitus if these factors apply. These epidemiology data reveal factors that are *correlated* with the presence of tinnitus and thus are not necessarily causative agents.

The most common risk factor for the onset of sensorineural tinnitus is noise exposure (Axelsson & Barrenas, 1992; Penner & Bilger, 1995). Also, a direct correlation exists between degree of hearing loss and prevalence of tinnitus—the odds of having tinnitus increase as hearing loss increases (Coles, 2000). This is true regardless of the type or the cause of the hearing loss. Dobie (2004b) concluded that tinnitus tends to occur more frequently in men, the elderly, blue-collar workers, and people with certain health problems.

Pathophysiology of Tinnitus

Many researchers are attempting to discover the pathophysiologic basis of tinnitus, with the ultimate goal of finding a cure for tinnitus. Numerous theories and models have been proposed; currently, there is no consensus regarding tinnitus mechanisms. It is beyond the scope of this book to go into detail regarding possible mechanisms of tinnitus generation. The interested reader is advised to review numerous excellent publications on this topic (e.g., Baguley, 2002; Eggermont, 2000; Kaltenbach, 2000; Møller, 2003; Tyler, 2006; Vernon & Møller, 1995). Because everything we hear (including tinnitus) results from neural activity in the auditory nervous system, tinnitus-mechanisms research has focused on understanding abnormal neural activity that is associated with tinnitus. Most theories involve hair cells, the auditory nerve, and the central auditory nervous system (J. A. Henry, Dennis, et al., 2005). A few examples of proposed mechanisms include (there are many others):

- *Hair cells:* discordant function between inner and outer hair cells (Jastreboff, 1990); damaged outer hair cells causing excessive release of neurotransmitter (glutamate) from inner hair cells producing sustained cochlear activity (Patuzzi, 2002).

- *Auditory nerve:* synchronization of spontaneous activity in auditory nerve fibers due to cross-talk (Eggermont, 1990; Møller, 1984, 1995); cortical reorganization following changes in the auditory periphery resulting in a disproportionately large number of neurons becoming sensitive (tuned) to frequencies at upper and lower borders representing peripheral hearing loss (Salvi, Lockwood, & Burkard, 2000).
- *Central auditory nervous system:* Increased spontaneous activity in the dorsal cochlear nucleus (Brozoski, Bauer, & Caspary, 2002; Kaltenbach & Afman, 2000; Kaltenbach et al., 2002; Zacharek, Kaltenbach, Mathog, & Zhang, 2002).

Data from Tinnitus Clinic Patients

Tinnitus Data Archive

The Oregon Health and Science University (OHSU) Tinnitus Clinic was started in 1975 (Vernon & Schleuning, 1978). Extensive data from thousands of patients have been collected, and these data have been used to develop the Tinnitus Data Archive (Meikle, Creedon, & Griest, 2004) (http://www.tinnitusarchive.org/). The summarized data in the Archive were collected from 1,630 patients seeking clinical intervention for their tinnitus and are not generalizable to individuals with tinnitus who do not seek intervention.

Main Findings of the Tinnitus Data Archive

Some of the main findings of the Tinnitus Data Archive include (J. A. Henry, Dennis, et al., 2005):

- There are about 2½ times more male than female patients.
- 80% of all patients are at least 40 years of age.
- Tinnitus onset is reported as "gradual" or "sudden" about equally.
- Left-sided tinnitus is reported more often than right-sided tinnitus.
- More than half of the patients describe their tinnitus as a single sound (most of the remainder identify two or more sounds).
- Most patients describe their tinnitus as "ringing" or "clear tone" (3% report "hum," "clicking," "roaring," or "pulse").
- 85% of patients indicated that their perceived tinnitus loudness was a 5 or more on a 0 to 10 loudness-rating scale (10 = "very loud").

Factors Associated with Tinnitus Onset

When OHSU Tinnitus Clinic patients were asked to describe the circumstances of their tinnitus onset, 43% indicated that no known events were associated. Most of the remainder reported that one factor was associated with their tinnitus onset (8% reported more than one factor).

For those patients describing factors associated with their tinnitus onset, the factors could be placed into one of four broad categories (Meikle et al., 2004): (1) noise-related; (2) head and neck trauma; (3) head and neck illness; and (4) other medical conditions.

Years "Aware of" Tinnitus

OHSU Tinnitus Clinic patients are asked how long they have been aware of experiencing tinnitus. From the Tinnitus Data Archive (Meikle et al., 2004), 40% of patients had experienced their tinnitus for 2 years or less; 55% for 5 years or less; 70% for 10 years or less; and 85% for 20 years or less.

Types of "Sounds" Patients Hear

Patients are asked to describe what their tinnitus sounds like from a list of sounds commonly reported by patients, or by describing a sound that is not on the list. The most common sound reported by far is "ringing." The second most common sound is "hissing." The third most common sound is "clear tone." Numerous additional sounds are reported, including "high-tension wire," "buzzing," "transformer noise," "sizzling," "crickets," "whistle," "hum," and "clicking."

Intermittency of Tinnitus

From the Tinnitus Data Archive, 91% of patients reported that their tinnitus is a constant sound. In 5% of patients, tinnitus is intermittent and heard more than 50% of the time. In 1% of patients, tinnitus is intermittent and heard less than 50% of the time.

Reduced Tolerance (Hypersensitivity) to Sound

"Hyperacusis" often is reported concurrently with tinnitus, and audiologists need to know how to recognize hyperacusis and how to provide appropriate intervention if it is a significant condition. There is no consensual definition of hyperacusis (P. J. Jastreboff & M. M. Jastreboff, 2004; Vernon, 2002). It has been defined as "the collapse of loudness tolerance so that almost all sounds produce loudness discomfort" (Vernon & Press, 1998). At the other extreme, clinics have reported that up to half of their patients experience decreased loudness tolerance (Coles, 1996; Gold, Frederick, & Formby, 1999; Hazell, 1999; P. J. Jastreboff, 2000). When evaluating the patient, the critical factor is to determine if loudness sensitivity is a significant problem in the patient's life.

Our definitions of conditions pertaining to decreased loudness tolerance are consistent with those published by J. A. Henry, Zaugg, and Schechter (2005a), which were adapted from P. J. Jastreboff and Hazell (2004).

Hyperacusis

Hyperacusis is a physical condition of discomfort or pain caused by sound. The effect is restricted primarily to the auditory pathways. Thus, a condition of "pure" hyperacusis causes physical discomfort, but no emotional responses are involved. For a given patient with pure hyperacusis, sound would be uncomfortably loud at levels most people find comfortable—*regardless of the type of sound*. This means that a patient who reports that he or she can tolerate some sounds at louder levels than other sounds is probably not experiencing pure hyperacusis.

Misophonia

M. M. Jastreboff and P. J. Jastreboff (2002) introduced the term misophonia. The term means "dislike of sound," and implies that there is an emotional reaction to sound. A misophonic reaction is a learned response. This means that a misophonic patient might report that a particular sound is problematic in some situations, but not in others. When questioned in detail, these patients often report reactions that would be inconsistent with pure hyperacusis. For example, they might report that certain "unpleasant" sounds become uncomfortably loud at levels below which "pleasant" sounds are tolerated comfortably.

Phonophobia

P. J. and M. M. Jastreboff (2000) defined use of the term phonophobia for clinical application. Phonophobia is a fear response caused by sound, and is considered a subcategory of misophonia. Misophonia can cause any kind of negative emotional response, but phonophobia specifically causes a fear reaction. A defining feature of phonophobia is the *anticipation* that sound will be uncomfortably loud. Thus, phonophobia refers to a person's state of mind with respect to sounds and sound environments.

Loudness Recruitment

Loudness recruitment often is confused with hyperacusis (Vernon, 2002). Recruitment refers to abnormally rapid growth in the perception of loudness (Vernon, 1976). It usually is a phenomenon of cochlear or sensorineural hearing loss. Recruitment generally is associated with reduced auditory thresholds and normal loudness discomfort levels (Figure 1–1). Thus, the dynamic range is compressed, but there is normal tolerance to louder sounds.

Treatment for Conditions of Reduced Sound Tolerance

In Chapter 6, we describe methodology for the treatment of reduced sound tolerance. The overall approach is to first determine if the condition is a severe problem for the patient. If so, then the patient should receive special treatment that focuses on the condition. If the condition is a mild or moderate problem, then the patient needs to be educated about the *sensitizing* effects of using hearing protection, and the *desensitizing* effects of using therapeutic sound (Formby & Gold, 2002). Normally, the use of sound that is advocated for tinnitus management will indirectly provide adequate treatment for reduced sound tolerance in mild and moderate cases. Consultation with a mental health provider might be useful if a patient fears sound and/or has other intense fears.

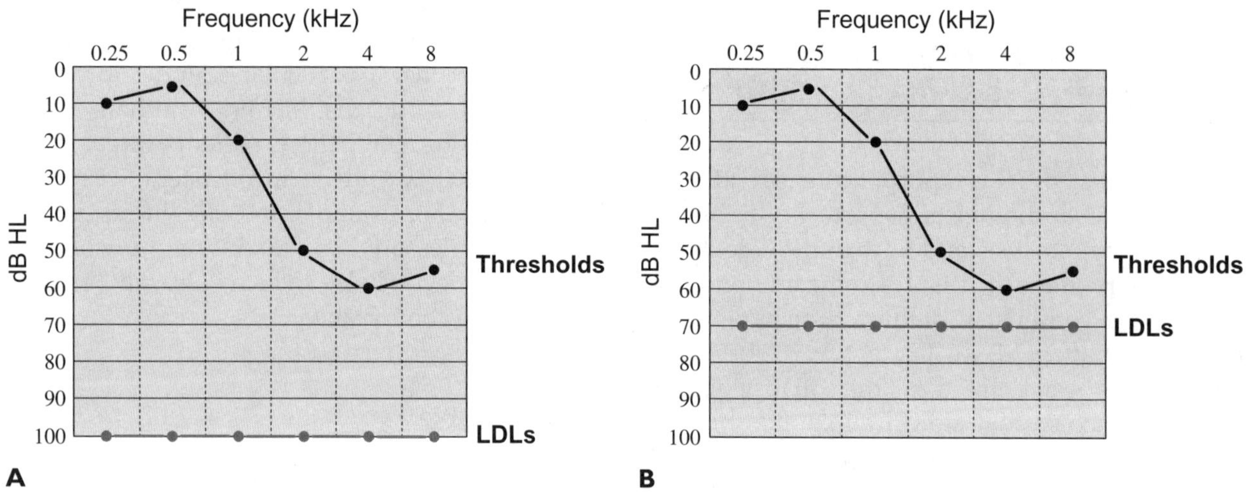

Figure 1–1. Tolerance to sound can be estimated by obtaining loudness discomfort levels (LDLs), which indicate the threshold level at which sound becomes uncomfortably loud. **A.** LDLs at and above about 100 dB HL are in the normal range. Note that the hearing sensitivity is reduced in the higher frequencies, resulting in a compressed dynamic range at those frequencies—and loudness recruitment. However, the LDLs at 100 dB HL reflect normal tolerance to louder sounds. **B.** LDLs are reduced to 70 dB HL, indicating a condition of reduced loudness tolerance. From *Tinnitus Retraining Therapy: Patient Counseling Guide* (p. 168), by J. A. Henry, D. R. Trune, M. J. A. Robb, & P. J. Jastreboff, 2007, San Diego, CA: Plural Publishing, Inc. Copyright 2007 by Plural Publishing. Reprinted with permission.

2

Research Leading to PTM

PTM

Progressive Tinnitus Management

In 2005, audiologic tinnitus management (ATM) was published as a comprehensive protocol for the management of tinnitus by audiologists (J. A. Henry, Zaugg, & Schechter, 2005a, 2005b). ATM was modified and expanded upon to create five hierarchical levels of clinical management, at which point the name was changed to "progressive" ATM (PATM) (J. A. Henry, Zaugg, Myers, & Schechter, 2008a, 2008b). PATM now is under revision to incorporate components of cognitive-behavioral therapy (CBT) to address psychological aspects of tinnitus (J. A. Henry, Zaugg, Myers, Kendall, & Turbin, 2009). As PATM is evolving to become inherently interdisciplinary, use of the word "audiologic" to describe the protocol no longer is appropriate. For that reason, the name was shortened to progressive tinnitus management (PTM).

The need for a *progressive* approach to tinnitus management became apparent as a result of conducting our series of controlled clinical studies. The PTM methodology evolved largely as a result of these experiences. Additional influences for PTM came from clinical experiences with patients and from consultation with experts from different disciplines whose insights in particular shaped the PTM patient education. PTM is designed to address the needs of all patients who complain about tinnitus while having minimal impact on clinical resources.

Prospective, controlled clinical studies are essential to evaluate and document the efficacy of tinnitus interventions. We have completed three studies and two are underway—both of which involve PTM. Conducting these studies required the development of highly specified protocols to ensure consistent performance of the various interventions. In addition, procedures were developed to efficiently screen and evaluate candidates to determine if they met study inclusion criteria, which differed for each study. Conducting these studies not only provided efficacy data, but also identified procedures that were most efficient for clinical application. Each of these studies and the insights gained from them are described below.

First Study

Our first study evaluated the relative efficacies of tinnitus masking (TM) and tinnitus retraining therapy (TRT) (J. A. Henry, Schechter, et al., 2006a, 2006b). For the study protocol, each of these methods involved the use of ear-level devices (hearing aids, noise generators, combination instruments) and intervention appointments at 0, 3, 6, 12, and 18 months. Only persons with very problematic tinnitus would warrant such rigorous, long-term clinical procedures. Therefore, it was necessary to carefully evaluate study candidates to determine their eligibility for receiving one of the interventions.

Advertising resulted in about 800 callers who expressed interest in participating. This level of response greatly exceeded our capacity to conduct a full clinical evaluation of each candidate. We therefore devised a three-stage screening protocol. For stage 1, a brief series of questions were administered to callers to establish that they experienced chronic tinnitus and that the tinnitus was so problematic that 18 months of intervention seemed justified. If so, they were invited for a hearing and tinnitus assessment (stage 2). Of the 800 callers, 171 (21%) received the stage 2 assessment. Following the assessment, those who qualified met with one of the tinnitus specialists (stage 3) to discuss results and to ensure a full understanding of all study requirements. Of the 171 who received the stage 3 assessment, 123 qualified and agreed to participate —representing only 15% of the original 800 callers.

Study outcomes were based on the Tinnitus Handicap Inventory (THI) (C. W. Newman, Jacobson, & Spitzer, 1996; C. W. Newman, Sandridge, & Jacobson, 1998). Overall, both TM and TRT cohorts showed significant improvement on the THI, with TRT providing greater benefit at 12 and 18 months (J. A. Henry, Schechter, et al., 2006a, 2006b).

Lessons Learned from First Study

The first study showed that both TM and TRT, when conducted in a tightly controlled manner, could provide significant benefit to a large majority of individuals with severely bothersome tinnitus. Both methods utilize broadband noise as therapeutic sound, but the application and purpose of the sound differ substantially between methods (J. A. Henry, Schechter, Nagler, & Fausti, 2002). With TM, sound is used to achieve an immediate sense of relief. "Immediate relief" is irrelevant with TRT because the objective of TRT is to create contrast reduction between tinnitus and the acoustic environment to promote habituation (P. J. Jastreboff, 2004). Our study provided evidence that these different clinical objectives largely were achieved for the two methods. Thus, a major lesson learned from this study was that sound can be used in different ways to accomplish different therapeutic objectives. The use of therapeutic sound with PTM expands on this concept to provide patients with an understanding of many different ways that sound can be used for tinnitus management. By understanding these different strategies for using sound, patients learn to use sound in a targeted manner to address any situation in which tinnitus is problematic.

With PTM, the basic strategies of using therapeutic sound with TM and TRT have been retained. However, the terminology and descriptions used with patients have been changed. These changes were designed to simplify the concepts for patients—to avoid misconceptions (such as thinking that the purpose of "masking" is to make the tinnitus inaudible) and to reduce confusion (such as trying to understand how specifically to achieve the "mixing point" with TRT). With PTM, use of sound to provide "immediate relief" is referred to as "soothing sound." Soothing sound can be used whenever patients wish to reduce stress or tension associated with tinnitus. Using sound to create "contrast reduction" is referred to as "background sound." Patients are advised to use background at all times as a passive-listening strategy to pay less attention to their tinnitus. Patients receiving PTM education learn to distinguish between the different applications of sound and to select different applications to accomplish different purposes.

For any clinical trial, it is necessary to determine if a candidate's condition warrants the intervention being offered. Our unexpectedly high volume of callers made it immediately evident that methodology was needed to provide efficient screening of individuals who claim to have a problem with tinnitus. In Chapter 3 we discuss how the large majority of people who experience tinnitus are not bothered by it. Many individuals with nonbothersome tinnitus, however, respond to announcements about tinnitus trials—even if the announcement states clearly that the study is for persons who are *bothered* by tinnitus. We needed methodology to query these callers to quickly assess the nature and severity of their tinnitus. It was particularly important to determine if a caller's complaint was due more to a hearing problem than to the tinnitus itself (J. A. Henry, Zaugg, et al., 2005a; Zaugg, Schechter, Fausti, & J. A. Henry, 2002). We have since developed and refined screening techniques to differentiate hearing problems from tinnitus problems. Most importantly, we developed the Tinnitus and Hearing Survey that now is the essential tool used with PTM for this purpose (see Chapter 5).

Second Study

The purpose of our second study was to determine the potential benefit of group education as intervention for bothersome tinnitus (J. A. Henry, Loovis, et al., 2007). The educational curriculum was an adaptation of the structured TRT counseling protocol. Participants attended four weekly 1.5-hour classes. Two control groups consisted of a "tinnitus support group" and a no-intervention group. The support group, also involving four weekly 1.5-hour meetings, was led by a facilitator who encouraged positive discussion about tinnitus but did not provide education. Veterans with bothersome tinnitus (n = 269) were randomized into one of the three groups. Outcomes were assessed at baseline and at 1, 6, and 12 months. Overall results revealed that group education provided significant improvement on the Tinnitus Severity Index (R. M. Johnson, 1998) from baseline through 12 months (p <.001). Neither of the control groups showed significant improvement from baseline to any of the follow-up time points.

Lessons Learned from Second Study

This study tested the effectiveness of a unique protocol of group education for tinnitus. Importantly, although participants did not receive an audiologic evaluation, 93% of the participants responded "sometimes," "usually," or "always" in response to the questionnaire item "Do you experience hearing difficulty?" In response to another item ("Does your tinnitus make it more difficult for you to hear?"), 83% responded "sometimes," "usually," or "always" (an additional 8% were "unsure"). In Chapters 3 and 5 we discuss the concern that many patients who complain about tinnitus mostly are bothered by hearing difficulties. Thus, when patients seek services for their tinnitus they may really need a hearing assessment and possibly hearing aids. Not addressing these participants' audiologic needs undoubtedly reduced the effectiveness of the group education. This insight confirmed the need to conduct a hearing evaluation and fit hearing aids if necessary as the first stage of management for tinnitus. For this reason, the Level 2 Audiologic Evaluation is the first stage of management with PTM, and includes a hearing evaluation and questionnaires to differentiate hearing problems from tinnitus-specific problems.

The benefit observed for the education group was sustained for 12 months, contrasting with results from a similar trial (J. L. Henry & P. H. Wilson, 1996). In that trial, significant improvement was observed on the Tinnitus Reaction Questionnaire for the education group immediately following the intervention, but which dissipated by 12 months. A major difference between the two education groups was that in our study the education group received focused instruction on using constant low-level background sound to facilitate habituation to tinnitus. It may be conjectured that the participants applied this information, thus facilitating the sustained benefit. Using constant background sound is a major instructional point with the PTM education and counseling.

Of the approximately 750 callers who were screened, 269 (36%) were enrolled. Thus, although all participants were offered the four education classes (those in the control groups could attend the classes after completing the study), 64% of the callers declined the opportunity to receive the education. Most callers indicated that their tinnitus was not enough of a problem to warrant attending the classes. This again speaks to the need to provide a hierarchy of clinical services so as to tailor services to the individual and to avoid providing more services than are necessary.

Additional insights gained from this study include: (a) a typical noneducational tinnitus support group does not seem to benefit the participants (thus, any group meetings for patients should include an appropriate educational component); and (b) individuals who are bothered by tinnitus but do not receive clinical services seem to stay at the same level with regard to how they are affected by their tinnitus (the fact that they don't seem to improve over a period of a year suggests that these individuals should receive clinical services). Most importantly, this study showed clear benefit of providing education in a group setting, which led to the development of PTM Level 3 Group Education (J. A. Henry, Zaugg, Myers, Kendall, et al., 2009).

Third Study

The first study evaluated the methods of TM and TRT to determine their efficacy for veterans who are severely bothered by tinnitus. Benefit was evident, but each method was conducted by an expert in the respective intervention. This third study was designed to determine if audiologists who are not tinnitus experts can provide effective intervention with TM and TRT. The study was conducted at four VA hospitals (Bay Pines, Florida; Portland, Oregon; San Diego, California; and Seattle, Washington). At each site, 36–38 veterans with clinically significant tinnitus (total $n = 148$) were recruited and randomized to TRT, TM, or a control group that received generic tinnitus counseling (i.e., nothing specific to TM or TRT) and hearing aids (if needed). Participants in all three groups received an initial evaluation and attended counseling appointments at 0, 3, 6, 12, and 18 months. Analyses revealed that each of the three groups showed significant improvement (based on mean index scores from the Tinnitus Handicap Inventory), with no significant differences between groups (publication in preparation).

Lessons Learned from Third Study

It was unexpected that the control group had outcomes comparable to TM and TRT. Although intended as a nonspecific-therapy control group, the counseling developed for this group was effective and subsequently published as part of the method referred to as audiologic tinnitus management (ATM) (J. A. Henry, Zaugg, et al., 2005b). The ATM counseling focused on how to use sound and sound-delivery devices to reduce the impact of tinnitus, which was the precursor to the counseling we have since developed for PTM. For PTM, these basic concepts have been refined and organized into a systematic description of the different ways that sound can be used to manage tinnitus. Thus, an insight from the third study was that a single approach to using sound may be too restrictive for addressing all of the different situations when tinnitus is problematic for patients. With PTM, patients are instructed in depth about the different uses of therapeutic sound to empower them to determine *on their own* how to use sound in a specific manner whenever their tinnitus is bothersome (J. A. Henry, Zaugg, Myers, Kendall, et al., 2009).

As a result of developing the "generic" counseling for the control group, we devised a third strategy for using therapeutic sound (in addition to using "soothing sound" and "background sound" as described under "Lessons Learned from First Study" above). The third strategy was to use sound for attention diversion, by listening to anything that would engage the mind for a sustained period. For PTM, this third strategy is referred to as using "interesting sound" with the purpose of focusing conscious attention away from the tinnitus and onto the target sound. Furthermore, the counseling created for the control group led to our development of numerous concepts, techniques, and tools for using therapeutic sound that now are described in the PTM self-help workbook and as part of the PTM educational counseling.

As for the first study, this third study required participants who were so bothered by their tinnitus that rigorous, long-term intervention was warranted. Screening methods that we developed as a result of the first and second studies were used with the third study to ensure that only qualified veterans were enrolled from the 505 candidates. Prior to completing all of the appointments, however, many participants realized that the intervention they had received was sufficient and that no further services were needed (30% of the participants dropped out of the study—most for this reason). Although it was gratifying to observe early therapeutic success, it was clear that a *progressive* approach was needed to provide services only to the degree necessary to meet individual needs. This progressive approach is a hallmark concept for PTM—patients undergo a series of short-term clinical interventions that can, if necessary, lead to Level 5 Individualized Support.

A comprehensive tinnitus assessment protocol was developed for use with all participants in this study. The protocol was published as one of the two ATM companion articles (J. A. Henry, Zaugg, et al., 2005a), and included: (a) a structured interview to identify problematic aspects of tinnitus; (b) a tinnitus psychoacoustic assessment; and (c) in-clinic trials to determine the potential benefit of ear-level noise generators and combination instruments. The protocol has since been refined for the PTM Level 4 Interdisciplinary Evaluation, and some components have been adapted for use during the Level 2 Audiologic Evaluation (J. A. Henry et al., 2008b).

Conducting this study required training 12 audiologists at four VA hospitals. The training was provided via the VA videoconferencing (V-Tel) system. Each study audiologist received about six hours of V-Tel training supplemented by a procedures manual. This training likely was inadequate for audiologists to perform methodology that normally requires much more training and considerable experience to attain a high level of proficiency. It was evident that any future tinnitus trials would require much more intensive training. For our pilot PTM study (described immediately below), we developed an extensive online training course as well as numerous clinical tools to facilitate all aspects of implementing the protocol.

Fourth Study

The fourth study currently is nearing completion at the James A. Haley Veterans' Hospital in Tampa, Florida. This study was designed to develop PTM and to evaluate its clinical efficacy in a pilot study to compare it to "usual care." Usual care (UC) involves services that are typical of what is provided at VA audiology clinics, that is, an audiologic examination, hearing aids if needed, and some minimal counseling specific to tinnitus. For this study, UC participants can receive ear-level noise generators or combination instruments if deemed necessary by the audiologist.

Development of the PTM implementation materials was a substantial undertaking requiring two years of continuous effort. Insights gained from our previous trials were applied to the PTM protocol. Five hierarchical levels of PTM were defined and detailed clinical procedures were developed for each level. A new counseling protocol was developed that incorporated principles of patient education and health literacy to ensure that the materials were accessible to as many patients as possible (J. A. Henry, Zaugg, Myers, Kendall, et al., 2009). An online, 18-module training course was developed for audiologists and numerous materials were developed for audiologists and patients. Major educational materials were developed to implement the protocol at the different levels.

As of November 2009, 221 clinical patients were enrolled by telephone in this study—109 were randomized to UC and 112 to PTM. Of these 221 patients, 21 who were randomized to UC, and 26 randomized to PTM, were excluded from study participation because they did not show up, called to be removed, or had a diagnosed psychotic disorder, dementia, or serious health concern. After excluding these 47 patients, 86 PTM patients and 88 UC patients attended an initial appointment and completed questionnaires. Of the 86 PTM patients, 23 attended at least one of the Level 3 Group Education sessions. Following Level 3, four patients attended a Level 4 evaluation. Only one PTM patient felt it was necessary to receive Level 5 Individualized Support. Of the 88 UC patients,

36 attended only the evaluation appointment and 52 attended a second appointment to receive hearing aids. As the study is still in progress, analyses of outcomes are not yet possible to determine how well patients do at the different levels of PTM.

Lessons Learned from Fourth Study

A major goal of this project was to learn about the process of putting the PTM protocol into clinical practice. To do so we conducted several formative evaluations. (A formative evaluation is "a rigorous assessment process designed to identify potential and actual influences on the progress and effectiveness of implementation efforts" [Stetler et al., 2006].) The results have been applied to our current research with PTM.

Online Course for Clinicians

An early, central element of implementing the PTM protocol is clinician education via an online course. The Chief of Audiology at the Tampa VA hospital made time available for each clinician to complete the 18-module course. All study audiologists completed the course and responded to embedded questions. These responses were compiled and analyzed to identify how to improve the course.

The online course currently is being revised and updated, and we are working with VA Employee Education System to make the course available via the VA Learning Management System (LMS). This course should become available for use by VA audiologists shortly after the publication of this handbook. We also will attempt to make the course available to non-VA audiologists.

When the online course becomes functional, an additional need will be to develop a program that simulates a clinical practicum for audiologists who have received the PTM training. To address this need, future plans include development of a "virtual clinic" to computer-simulate patients receiving clinical services with PTM. The program will depict patients with a variety of clinical presentations and clinicians will be challenged to make appropriate decisions to provide optimal care.

Conference Calls Held with PTM Audiologists

During these calls with clinicians and the study team, semistructured discussions addressed the acceptance and general satisfaction with the protocol as well as any difficulties performing each level of PTM care. Notes from these calls were compiled and reviewed to identify any barriers or facilitators to the management of tinnitus using PTM. We are adapting the program to be responsive to the feedback received from these calls.

Clinical Implementation of PTM

By collecting formative data during the implementation of PTM in the Tampa VA Audiology Clinic, we learned that preplanning for some of the activities could improve the implementation process. For example, prior to starting the program, administrators should know that (a) the PTM audiologists will require release time to complete the Web-course; (b) the audiologists will be working with psychologists, which will require preplanning with the psychology section of the hospital; (c) patients being seen for tinnitus will need hearing evaluations and may need ear-level devices; and (d) the PTM protocol necessitates access by audiologists to a meeting room for the Level 3 workshops. We also recommend holding regular calls or meetings with audiologists who are beginning to use the protocol to address barriers that may arise as they put PTM into practice. Valuable information can be identified and acted on to improve fidelity to protocol.

Patients in this pilot study were all veterans at the Tampa VA hospital who complained of bothersome tinnitus. As all of the patients in the PTM cohort were offered tinnitus services beyond Level 2 Audiologic Evaluation, it is clear that the majority of these patients either chose not to receive higher-level services or it was too difficult for them to attend the additional visits that were required to participate in the Level 3 workshops. We will look carefully at the data to determine if patients' perceptions of adequate care following Level 2 are accurate. We now are more strongly advising patients to attend Level 3 Group Education to ensure that each patient who is bothered by tinnitus receives the education that is essential to learn basic self-management skills. We also provided patients in the PTM cohort the self-help workbook at the end of Level 2. We now are recommending that the workbook not be provided to patients until they attend their first Level 3 workshop (see Chapters 3 and 5).

Finally, only a few patients in the PTM cohort required services beyond Level 3. With the addition of CBT to the Level 3 protocol, the effectiveness of the Level 3 workshops is expected to be substantially improved, which should ensure that very few patients will require Level 4 and 5 services.

Fifth Study

This is an observational pilot study currently being conducted to assess an adaptation of the PTM methodology for use with veterans and active military who have experienced traumatic brain injury (TBI) and also have bothersome tinnitus. As these individuals are located all over the country, we developed a home-based telehealth method. The procedures are conducted over the telephone, and intervention materials and questionnaires are delivered via the mail/FedEx. The study includes three cohorts (all with bothersome tinnitus): (a) probable mild TBI history; (b) moderate or severe TBI; and (c) no TBI.

Interested callers are screened for tinnitus severity and probable TBI history. Callers who pass screening are sent the self-help workbook (2nd edition prepared specifically for this study) along with baseline questionnaires and the informed consent form. The research coordinator then conducts informed consent, assesses "capacity" (cognitive ability) for candidates to provide informed consent, and enrolls eligible candidates. Participants attend a telephone appointment with the study psychologist who conducts brief cognitive screening and teaches coping techniques for managing reactions to tinnitus based on CBT (J. L. Henry & P. H. Wilson, 2001). The next appointment is with the study audiologist who provides the PTM audiologic/sound-based counseling that normally is provided at Level 3 Group Education, but in a one-on-one format similar to Level 5 Individualized Support (J. A. Henry, Zaugg, Myers, Kendall, et al., 2009). Telephone appointments alternate between the psychologist and audiologist for 6 months (total of seven appointments).

As of November 2009, 172 individuals called about the study. Of these, 36 participants were enrolled, including 15 in the probable-mild TBI group, 10 in the moderate/severe TBI group, and 11 in the no-TBI group. Twelve-week outcome data are available for 23 participants, and 24-week outcome data are available for 16 participants. Preliminary results of the primary outcomes can be summarized as follows. On average, participants lowered their Baseline THI scores by 13.6 points at the 12-week evaluation, and by 21.7 points at 24 weeks. Because outcome data are incomplete, and because of the small numbers of participants, these data cannot yet be subjected to statistical comparisons.

Lessons Learned from Fifth Study

This project responds to the need to provide special clinical services for veterans and military personnel who have experienced TBI and also suffer from bothersome tinnitus. Because of the complications of TBI, it was necessary to include a neuropsychologist with expertise in TBI and a clinical psychologist with expertise in tinnitus management to assist in the design and implementation of the trial. These collaborators have made the necessary revisions to the PTM protocol so that it is appropriate for telephone-based administration to TBI patients. For example, the participants undergo a cognitive screen to determine their abilities to comprehend the counseling information and to follow through with the management recommendations.

Prior to the design and development of this study, it was obvious that psychological concerns were not adequately addressed by the PTM counseling. This was a shortcoming that is being addressed for the first time using the PTM protocol in this pilot study. The PTM protocol thus is evolving to include counseling that covers all aspects of using therapeutic sound as well as addressing psychological components of tinnitus. Several researchers have conducted clinical trials that support CBT as an effective psychological method for managing tinnitus (Martinez Devesa, Waddell, Perera, & Theodoulou, 2007). Thus, CBT was incorporated into the PTM method. The components of CBT that are being used include training in behavioral modification (stress management via relaxation techniques and scheduling pleasant activities), as well as cognitive restructuring (step-by-step examination of changing thoughts to acquire a more positive attitude about tinnitus). Thus, abbreviated telephone-based CBT was developed to incorporate essential features of this psychotherapy.

The addition of CBT to the PTM protocol required expansion of the self-help workbook to include the new information. We developed a second edition of the workbook that is mailed to all participants in this pilot study (J. A. Henry, Zaugg, Myers, & Kendall, 2009). This new workbook also contains two DVDs that supplement the written material: (a) interactive video that guides patients through the material normally presented in PTM Level 3 Group Education; and (b) demonstrations of relaxation training exercises including deep breathing and imagery. We recently completed the third edition of the workbook based on feedback from subjects using it during this pilot study, which is being distributed to all VA audiologists and also is in publication for non-VA use (J. A. Henry, Zaugg, Myers, & Kendall, 2010a). The workbook contains a DVD and CD that were developed through VA Employee Education System.

Additional Evidence Supporting PTM

Numerous studies have supported the use of therapeutic sound for tinnitus management. Evidence has been provided by these studies supporting the beneficial use of: (a) hearing aids (Del Bo & Ambrosetti, 2007; Folmer & Carroll, 2006; Saltzman & Ersner, 1947; Surr, Kolb, Cord, & Garrus, 1999; Surr, Montgomery, & Mueller, 1985; Trotter & Donaldson, 2008); (b) ear-level masking devices (Folmer & Carroll, 2006; Hazell et al., 1985; Schleuning, Johnson, & Vernon, 1980; Stephens & Corcoran, 1985); (c) TRT (Bartnik, Fabijanska, & Rogowski, 2001; Berry, Gold, Frederick, Gray, & Staecker, 2002; Herraiz, Hernandez, Plaza, & de los Santos, 2005; Herraiz, Hernandez, Toledano, & Aparicio, 2007); and (d) neuromonics tinnitus treatment (P. B. Davis, Paki, & Hanley, 2007). Our first clinical study (see First Study above) demonstrated that all types of ear-level devices (hearing aids, sound generators, and combination instruments) could be used effectively with both TM and TRT (J. A. Henry, Schechter, et al., 2006a, 2006b). Our third clinical study (see Third Study above) extended the first clinical trial and showed that TM, TRT, and a nonspecific control group all provide significant benefit to subjects. Folmer and Carroll (2006) evaluated 150 patients who attended a comprehensive tinnitus management clinic, including patients who (a) used hearing aids ($n = 50$); (b) used ear-level noise generators ($n = 50$); and (c) did not use ear-level devices ($n = 50$). Significant improvement was experienced by all three groups. Notably, the patients who used hearing aids and noise generators experienced significantly greater benefit than did the patients who did not receive devices.

As a whole, these many studies comprise a strong body of support for the efficacy of using therapeutic sound to manage tinnitus. It should be noted, however, that the evidence does not demonstrate that any one of these methods is superior to any other. Rather, it appears that any judicious use of sound seems to be helpful for managing tinnitus, and it may be that some methods are more helpful in certain situations and for certain patients. Clearly, research is needed that systematically evaluates the different parameters of sound to determine which parameters provide the greatest benefit and under what conditions. With PTM, the overriding philosophy is that therapeutic sound provides the greatest benefit when patients are informed about the different uses of sound for tinnitus management, and when patients learn how to develop, on their own, sound-management plans to address specific situations when their tinnitus is problematic. PTM utilizes procedures that encourage patients to incorporate good self-management practices.

CBT is an evidence-based and appropriate addition to PTM to address the psychological components of tinnitus distress that are so common with these patients. CBT is a type of psychotherapy that targets specific thoughts, core beliefs, and negative appraisals of situations that are unconstructive (and may cause distress) while providing tools for implementing more adaptive behavioral and cognitive modifications (Beck, 1995; Sweetow, 2000). Martinez Devesa et al. (2007) conducted a meta-analysis of six randomized, controlled studies (285 participants) of CBT for tinnitus. They found significant improvement in quality of life (decrease of global tinnitus severity) for those receiving CBT compared to those who did not receive CBT.

Summary

The five levels of PTM provide a logical, sequential means of working collaboratively with a patient to best determine the patient's needs and to provide only the services that are needed. PTM patients receive only basic audiology services and tinnitus education (from an audiologist and a psychologist) through Level 3, which do not require a major commitment on the part of either the clinician or the patient. Included in the education are thorough explanations of the different ways that therapeutic sound and coping skills can be used to manage reactions to tinnitus. Patients are then taught how other sound-based methods use therapeutic sound. Patients should have this understanding before committing to an expensive and time-consuming clinical protocol. This also is the reason that fitting ear-level noise generators or combination instruments is not normally advocated until Level 4. Patients need to be fully informed before making such consequential decisions.

Tinnitus research has been conducted at the Portland VA Medical Center since 1995 (under the auspices of the NCRAR since 1997). In 1999 we began a series of clinical trials to evaluate different methods of tinnitus management, which provided the experience and data that led to development of the PTM model of care. The basic content of the PTM protocol (i.e., the levels of care) has been defined from the results of our years of research. The addition of CBT techniques to the PTM protocol addresses psychological aspects of tinnitus and thereby is expected to improve the effectiveness of PTM. The basic PTM protocol continues to provide a framework for "progressive" management for clinical expediency, but the clinical services provided now are of a more interdisciplinary nature.

3

Overview of PTM

PTM

Progressive Tinnitus Management

In this chapter, we provide an overview of progressive tinnitus management (PTM). We start by describing basic principles that undergird the PTM protocol. We then provide summaries of each of the different levels of PTM, followed by case studies that exemplify the individualized nature of providing hierarchical services with PTM.

Basic Premises for PTM

Manage Reactions to Tinnitus

Chronic tinnitus (as distinct from somatosounds) reflects malfunction somewhere within the auditory system. The phantom perception of sound is a symptom of the malfunction. Normally, the malfunction cannot be corrected and intervention cannot permanently reduce the loudness/intensity of the symptom. Considering that reducing the loudness of tinnitus normally is not an option, the next best thing is to help patients live more comfortably with their tinnitus. The focus of PTM is to teach patients how to *manage their reactions* to tinnitus, which can make a meaningful difference in quality of life.

What do we mean by "manage reactions" to tinnitus? Note that we avoid the word "treatment," which might be interpreted by patients to mean that a circumscribed course of treatment will permanently quiet or eliminate their tinnitus. Such an outcome typically is what patients want, and they often are not interested in receiving clinical services if those services will not cure their tinnitus. Patients need to be informed that although tinnitus cannot be cured they can learn to manage their reactions to it, thereby improving their quality of life.

Any reference to "managing tinnitus" really means "managing *reactions* to tinnitus." "Managing tinnitus" might be misinterpreted to mean "managing the sound of tinnitus" or "doing something to make the tinnitus quieter." Because we cannot change tinnitus itself, tinnitus management should be interpreted to mean making lifestyle adjustments to reduce any reactions to tinnitus. "Reactions" pertains to any negative effects of tinnitus on quality of life, such as sleep disturbance, concentration difficulties, or any negative emotions that are associated with tinnitus.

By learning to self-manage their reactions to tinnitus, patients are empowered by gaining the ability to know how to address any situation in which their tinnitus is bothersome or intrusive. Patients need varying levels of support and guidance from providers before becoming self-sufficient in this process. Thus, there is a level of participation required of patients—they are expected to be engaged in the "collaborative self-management" process (J. A. Henry, Zaugg, Myers, Kendall, et al., 2009) until they are able to independently manage their reactions to tinnitus (see Chapter 7).

Intervention with PTM specifically involves activities designed to reduce reactions to tinnitus (no attempt is made to alter the tinnitus sound). In addition, patients with tinnitus are taught basic concepts of hearing conservation. Learning these concepts is universally important and is particularly necessary for anyone who experiences tinnitus to minimize the potential for exacerbation of the tinnitus symptom.

Clinical Services Should Be Progressive

As mentioned in Chapter 1, epidemiologic studies reveal that chronic tinnitus is experienced by about 10 to 15% of all adults (H. J. Hoffman & Reed, 2004). However, the condition is "clinically significant" for only about 20% of those who experience tinnitus (A. Davis & Refaie, 2000; P. J. Jastreboff & Hazell, 1998).

Tinnitus that is "clinically significant" indicates that the tinnitus causes functional impairment to such a degree that clinical intervention is warranted. Although difficult to define, some criterion level of functional impairment would categorize an individual as requiring clinical intervention. Determining this criterion level must be based on the person's perception of the need for intervention. As a general guide, tinnitus is likely to be clinically significant if the person agrees with each of the following statements:

- The tinnitus disrupts at least one important life activity.
- The degree of disruption is "more than trivial."
- The disruption causes a noticeable reduction in quality of life.
- The benefit from intervention would outweigh the cost and effort (i.e., "the effort would be worth it").

The "tinnitus pyramid" (Figure 3–1) depicts how individuals who experience tinnitus are distributed with respect to how the tinnitus impacts their lives (Dobie, 2004b). The pyramid shows that the majority of these people either are not bothered by it or they require only some basic education. Approaching the top of the pyramid are people who have progressively more severe problems caused by tinnitus. The top contains the relatively few patients who are "debilitated" by their tinnitus.

Most patients do not require extensive (or expensive) clinical intervention to learn how to manage their reactions to tinnitus. We therefore developed a hierarchical approach to efficiently provide clinical services to patients having diverse levels of need. Figure 3–2 shows the five levels of PTM, which are described in detail as the primary focus of this book.

The observation that the majority of individuals who experience tinnitus do not require intervention has been supported by numerous subject-recruitment efforts for controlled studies conducted at the Portland VA Medical Center (under the auspices of the National Center for Rehabilitative Auditory Research, NCRAR) to evaluate methods of tinnitus intervention (see Chapter 2). For each study, we are contacted by large numbers of individuals who are interested in participating. However, just *experiencing* tinnitus is not justification for receiving therapy that is designed to address *reactions* to tinnitus. As explained in Chapter 2, we had to develop screening methodology to determine *if* a person requires intervention. Furthermore, individuals who do require intervention have different levels of need, ranging from brief counseling to individualized, ongoing therapy—thus the rationale for *progressive* clinical services.

The overall goal of the hierarchical approach used with PTM is to minimize the impact of tinnitus on patients' lives as efficiently as possible. The model is designed to be maximally efficient to have the least impact on clinical resources, while still addressing the needs of all patients who complain of tinnitus.

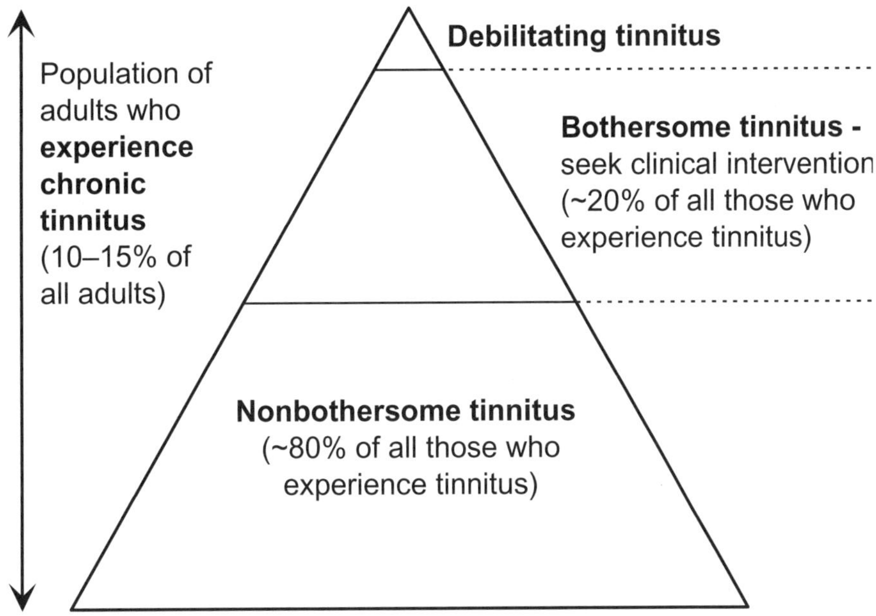

Figure 3–1. The Tinnitus Pyramid (Dobie, 2004b). The concept depicted here is that the pyramid contains the entire population of people who experience chronic tinnitus. The majority of these people (in the lower part of the pyramid) are not particularly bothered by their tinnitus. Many of these people only want assurance that their tinnitus does not reflect some serious medical condition (those in the middle of the pyramid). Relatively few have tinnitus that requires some degree of clinical intervention (toward the top of the pyramid). A very small fraction has "debilitating" tinnitus (in the top of the pyramid).

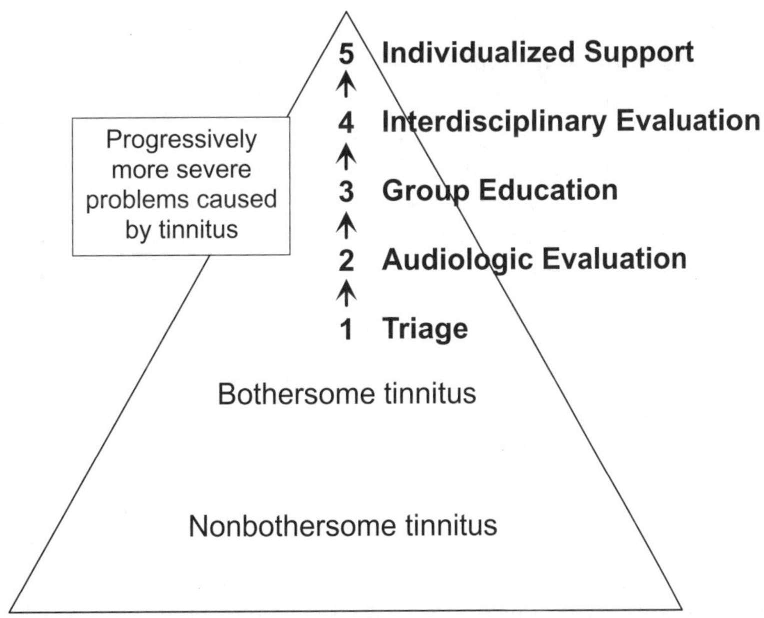

Figure 3–2. Five levels of progressive tinnitus management (PTM) superimposed on the Tinnitus Pyramid (see Figure 3–1). Each higher level reflects a greater intensity of clinical services, and patients progress only to the level needed.

Use an Interdisciplinary Approach

The initial evaluation for a patient who complains of tinnitus usually can be conducted by an audiologist and in many cases the audiology assessment (with the possibility of fitting hearing aids) is the only service needed. However, many patients require referral for additional evaluations, and some patients require tinnitus-specific intervention. Because of the multiple dimensions of problematic tinnitus, clinical services are optimized by using an interdisciplinary approach.

Clinical evaluations help determine the range and types of services needed to manage the full scope of medical, rehabilitation, and psychosocial aspects of tinnitus. Members of the tinnitus management team administer a variety of assessment instruments and then, for difficult cases, meet as a group to integrate results into a plan of care tailored to the individual needs of the patient. The scope of care depends on the severity of perceived tinnitus and medical and psychological issues. Intervention for tinnitus typically requires audiology and mental health services but may involve medical and prosthetic services.

Audiologist

Audiologists are essential for providing clinical services for tinnitus (J. A. Henry, Zaugg, et al., 2005a). Although audiologists can independently perform all aspects of clinical services for many patients, it is vital that they refer patients to other health care professionals as the presenting symptoms warrant. Audiologists must be aware of certain tinnitus-specific symptoms that indicate the need for medical evaluation services. Audiologists also must be aware of symptoms consistent with medical and psychological conditions. Optimally, audiologists who provide tinnitus services should work with an interdisciplinary tinnitus team.

Physician Ear Specialist

Ideally, every patient complaining of tinnitus would receive a complete head and neck examination from an otolaryngologist, otologist, or neuro-otologist who is knowledgeable about the multiple causes and presentations of tinnitus. However, this is not practical or realistic in many cases. Guidelines are provided in Chapters 4, 5, and 8 for determining when a medical evaluation is necessary. For example, pulsatile tinnitus often has an identifiable site, for which there are many potential causes. All patients who present with pulsatile tinnitus should receive a medical evaluation—primarily to rule out pathology (e.g., glomus tumor) that requires medical intervention.

Mental Health Professional

Some patients with tinnitus present with behaviors that indicate the need for an evaluation by a psychiatrist, psychologist, or other licensed mental health professional. Most mental/emotional disorders are not so obvious and require special evaluations to establish their existence and significance. A relatively high proportion of patients concerned about tinnitus suffer from depression and/or anxiety (Dobie, 2003; Halford & Anderson, 1991; Kirsch, Blanchard, & Parnes, 1989). Patients suspected of having these problems should be referred for evaluation by a mental health professional. Patients also should be referred immediately to a mental health professional if they report suicidal or violent thoughts, or if they report bizarre symptoms such as "hearing voices."

Tinnitus can be associated with post-traumatic stress disorder (PTSD). PTSD is a constellation of mental, emotional, and physical symptoms that can follow the experience of a traumatic event. Although commonly associated with military veterans, PTSD affects all strata of the population and all manner of psychological trauma. Untreated PTSD can impede rehabilitation efforts, including the clinical management of tinnitus. Failure to properly refer patients for possible PTSD, depression, and/or chronic anxiety reduces the likelihood of achieving the desired outcomes from tinnitus intervention.

Sleep disturbance is the nonauditory problem most frequently reported by patients with tinnitus (Erlandsson, 2000; Jakes, Hallam, Chambers, & Hinchcliffe, 1985; Meikle & Walsh, 1984; Tyler & Baker, 1983). Patients who report sleep problems also tend to have the most severe tinnitus. Sleep problems may be mitigated by teaching sleep-management techniques that are included in both the psychologic and audiologic portions of the PTM counseling (and in the PTM self-help workbook). If these efforts are not successful, then the patient may need referral to a sleep disorders specialist, physician, or mental health professional.

Prosthetics

Some aspects of PTM incorporate instruments including hearing aids, ear-level noise generators ("maskers") and combination instruments (combined hearing aid and masker), as well as wearable and tabletop devices that are used for sound therapy purposes. Involvement of prosthetics and sensory aids staff (at VA, military, and some other hospitals and clinics) ensures that appropriate technology will be available to patients with tinnitus.

Start with Audiologic Assessment

Patients complaining of tinnitus need an audiologic assessment for two basic reasons. First, they must be evaluated to determine if referral to a physician is warranted. Second, tinnitus usually is associated with some degree of hearing loss (Axelsson & Ringdahl, 1989; A. Davis & Refaie, 2000; J. L. Henry & P. H. Wilson, 2001; Vernon, 1998). Our research has revealed that the great majority of patients who complain of tinnitus also complain of hearing problems (J. A. Henry, Loovis, et al., 2007). An audiologic examination should be the clinical starting point for all patients who complain of tinnitus, unless urgent medical services are required.

In addition to the audiology testing, a brief assessment should be performed to determine if intervention specific to tinnitus is warranted. Patients with tinnitus commonly (and erroneously) attribute hearing problems to tinnitus (Coles, 1995; Dobie, 2004b; Zaugg et al., 2002). It therefore is critical to determine how much of the patient's complaint is due to a hearing problem and how much is due specifically to the tinnitus. PTM utilizes a brief questionnaire (Tinnitus and Hearing Survey—see Chapter 5) to help make this determination.

Focus on Patient Education as Intervention

Clinical intervention with PTM relies on a structured program of patient education. The education consists primarily of teaching patients how to use sound and coping techniques to manage their reactions to tinnitus. More specifically, patients learn how to develop and implement individualized plans for using therapeutic sound and apply principles of cognitive-behavioral therapy (CBT) to manage their tinnitus. Success in achieving these goals depends largely upon patients acquiring confidence in applying the self-management strategies. Breaking the process of learning how to manage tinnitus into small achievable tasks helps to ensure that patients experience initial success. This approach is in accordance with the self-efficacy theory (Bandura, 1977). Research has demonstrated that self-efficacy is a good predictor of motivation and behavior. In general, the experience of success increases self-efficacy while experiencing failure reduces self-efficacy.

Unique aspects of intervention with PTM include: (a) its emphasis on collaborative management by patient and clinician, leading to self-management by the patient; (b) development and use of sound-based therapy that is customized to address patients' individual needs; (c) application of evidence-based principles of patient education and health literacy; (d) use of multiple modalities to provide education within different levels of PTM; and (e) inclusion of essential components of CBT to teach coping skills (J. A. Henry, Zaugg, Myers, Kendall, et al., 2009).

PTM education is provided to patients at Levels 2, 3, and 5, but in a different format at each of these levels. Going from lower to higher levels the education becomes increasingly more personalized. At Level 2, patients can receive the self-management workbook (although it is recommended to give the workbook to patients at the start of Level 3 intervention). The workbook contains step-by-step instructions for patients to learn the self-management techniques on their own. All patients with tinnitus-specific problems are advised to participate in the workshops that comprise Level 3 Group Education. At Level 5, the education is provided in a one-on-one format.

The Audiologist's Role as Patient Educator

Patient education is the most important aspect of providing intervention with PTM. Thus, one of the audiologist's primary roles in this program is that of patient educator. Training received by audiologists generally does not include theories and concepts of patient education for achieving changes in behavior. We previously have published a description of the principles of education used with PTM (J. A. Henry, Zaugg, Myers, Kendall, et al., 2009). The information in that article can help audiologists better understand their role as patient educator and maximize their effectiveness in implementing the educational components of PTM.

Address the Problem of Low Health Literacy

Nearly one third of English-speaking adults in the United States have low health literacy (Gazmararian et al., 1999; Nielsen-Bohlman, Panzer, & Kindig, 2004; Williams et al., 1995). Those with low health literacy have an incomplete understanding of their health problems, and are more likely to report poor health, have more hospitalizations and higher health care costs, as well as suffer worse health outcomes overall (Baker, Parker, Williams, Clark, & Nurss, 1997; Howard, Gazmararian, & Parker, 2005; Weiss, Hart, McGee, & D'Estelle, 1992; Weiss & Palmer, 2004). Tinnitus disproportionately affects the populations most likely to have low health literacy: older adults and low-income individuals (S. C. Brown, 1990; Doak, Doak, & Root, 1996; Heller, 2003; H. J. Hoffman & Reed, 2004; Sindhusake, Mitchell, et al., 2003).

Even literate persons may have difficulty understanding health information, so training clinicians to communicate in ways that reach low-literate patients is good for all patients (Mayeaux et al., 1996). There is general consensus among health literacy and communication experts that the seven strategies we have described previously (J. A. Henry, Zaugg, Myers, Kendall, et al., 2009) can help improve provider-patient communication (Doak et al., 1996; Williams, Davis, Parker, & Weiss, 2002). These strategies are incorporated into the PTM educational and counseling materials and should be adopted during all interactions with patients.

Refer Patients Appropriately

Because tinnitus can be a multidimensional problem, a team approach is the ideal. The team approach, however, currently is seen in very few clinics. Therefore, it is vitally important that patients are referred as appropriate to other health care professionals. Ideally, PTM services will be a joint effort between audiology and psychology, with inclusion of otolaryngology, psychiatry, and other disciplines as needed. Mental health professionals who receive tinnitus referrals should have expertise in providing psychological interventions for patients with chronic health conditions and at least be familiar with the nature of tinnitus within the context of comorbid psychological problems.

Five Levels of PTM

Synopsis

The PTM Flowchart (Appendix A) shows the five hierarchical levels of clinical services with PTM. The hierarchy of services starts with Level 1 Triage at the bottom of the flowchart. Level 1 Triage provides guidelines for all clinics where patients with tinnitus are likely to be encountered. Level 1 Triage on the flowchart includes a large rectangular text box that describes the criteria for referring patients who complain of tinnitus. Depending on the patient's symptoms and other diagnostic factors, there are four possible referrals (as indicated by the four columns in the text box): (1) Refer to audiology; (2) Refer to ENT (i.e., refer to otolaryngology) for a nonurgent appointment; (3) Refer to emergency care or ENT for an urgent appointment that will take place on the same day the symptoms are reported; (4) Refer to mental health or emergency care for further assessment of concerning mental health symptoms.

Level 2 of PTM is the Audiologic Evaluation, during which it is determined whether or not the patient will participate in Level 3 Group Education. During the Level 2 evaluation, patients also are screened for severely reduced tolerance to sound (hyperacusis). If they fail the screening, then they should participate in the sound tolerance evaluation and management (STEM) protocol, as indicated on the figure. The STEM protocol should resolve the hyperacusis problem, at which time the patient should be evaluated to determine if further tinnitus services are needed. If so, then the patient is advised to participate in Level 3 Group Education (shown on the flowchart by the arrow leading from the STEM box to Level 3).

Patients who need clinical services beyond Level 3 can schedule an appointment for a Level 4 Interdisciplinary Evaluation. The Level 4 evaluation (ideally performed by an audiologist and a psychologist) will be used to determine if Level 5 Individualized Support is warranted.

Level I Triage

> **Level 1** is the **triage** level for referring patients at the initial clinic point-of-contact.

"Tinnitus triage guidelines" were developed for nonaudiologist health care providers who encounter patients complaining of tinnitus. Patients complain of tinnitus in many different clinical settings. Health care providers often do not know how to refer these patients appropriately—or whether to refer them at all. The tinnitus triage guidelines can be used to help guide referral practices for clinicians encountering patients reporting tinnitus. The guidelines are consistent with accepted clinical practices (Harrop-Griffiths, Katon, Dobie, Sakai, & Russo, 1987; J. A. Henry, Zaugg, et al., 2005a; J. L. Henry & P. H. Wilson, 2001; Wackym & Friedland, 2004).

Level 2 Audiologic Evaluation

> **Level 2** is the **audiologic evaluation**, which includes a brief assessment of the impact of tinnitus on the patient's life.

The primary objective of the Level 2 Audiologic Evaluation is to assess the potential need for a medical examination and/or audiologic intervention (audiologic intervention can include intervention for hearing loss, tinnitus, and/or reduced sound tolerance). Sometimes it also is appropriate to screen for mental health conditions that can interfere with successful self-management of reactions to tinnitus. Screening methodology is available, but not required, at this level to determine if a patient should be referred for a mental health assessment. When indicated, brief questionnaires can be administered to assess the potential need for referral to a mental health clinic. Patients' primary care providers should be notified when their patients report feeling sad, isolated, agitated, or anxious. This information should be documented in the medical record along with behavioral observations such as crying or angry outbursts.

The Level 2 evaluation always includes a standard audiologic evaluation and brief written questionnaires to assess the relative impact of hearing problems and tinnitus problems. Patients who require amplification are fitted with hearing aids, which often can result in satisfactory reduction in reactions to tinnitus with minimal education and support specific to tinnitus (J. A. Henry, Zaugg, Myers, & Schechter, 2008c; J. A. Henry, Zaugg, et al., 2005b; Searchfield, 2005). Patients who report any degree of a tinnitus problem following these basic services are advised to attend Level 3 Group Education.

Patients who report a severe problem with reduced sound tolerance are scheduled for STEM, which then becomes the focus of clinical management. (STEM is described fully in Chapter 6, and a brief summary is provided below.)

Patient Self-Help Workbook

> The **self-help workbook** provides a description of key information that is covered during Level 3 Group Education.

A special workbook (*How to Manage Your Tinnitus: A Step-by-Step Workbook*) (J. A. Henry et al., 2010a) has been developed that provides patients with the core PTM counseling information that is offered both in Level 3 Group Education and Level 5 Individualized Support. The workbook provides detailed information and instructions for developing individualized action plans to self-manage reactions to tinnitus using therapeutic sound and coping techniques. Videos and a sound demonstration CD are included in the workbook to supplement the written material.

Although the workbook is designed to be used by patients to learn the different self-help techniques, it has been our experience that many patients have difficulty benefiting from the workbook without at least some guidance and support from a clinician. Indeed, some patients can receive full benefit from using the workbook without additional intervention. However, patients are more likely to benefit from the workbook if it is provided in the context of a group with guided activities led by a clinician. We recommend providing the workbook to patients when they attend their first Level 3 workshop—for reasons that are explained in Chapter 5.

Sound Tolerance Evaluation and Management (STEM)

STEM provides adjunct procedures to **evaluate and treat a severe sound tolerance problem.**

During the Level 2 Audiologic Evaluation, patients are screened for a sound tolerance problem (hyperacusis and/or misophonia) using the Tinnitus and Hearing Survey (see Chapter 5). The survey includes two questions specific to reduced sound tolerance, which generally are adequate to determine if the patient has a severe problem with reduced sound tolerance. These patients are considered special cases and their progress through PTM is temporarily suspended while they undergo STEM. Some patients also may express a strong desire to simply concentrate on addressing sound tolerance problems rather than tinnitus. These patients should have the option of attending the STEM program.

The STEM protocol starts with an assessment of the problem, which relies mainly upon a special sound tolerance interview (see Chapter 6). Testing for loudness discomfort levels can be performed, but is not required. If treatment for reduced sound tolerance is needed, then the use of ear-level devices (noise generators or combination instruments) is a consideration. Special procedures have been developed to evaluate patients for these devices. The STEM protocol continues for as long as reduced sound tolerance is a significant problem for the patient. Once the sound tolerance problem is under control, then it is determined whether the patient should continue to receive tinnitus-specific clinical services. If so, then the patient normally is advised to participate in Level 3 Group Education.

Level 3 Group Education

Level 3 provides **group education workshops** for patients who require tinnitus-specific intervention.

Level 3 Group Education is for patients who have attended the Level 2 Audiologic Evaluation and feel that they need additional clinical services to learn how to manage their reactions to tinnitus. Level 3 is the first level within PTM for which patients receive focused intervention for a tinnitus problem. The group education is presented as classroom-style sessions of PTM counseling that are facilitated by the use of PowerPoint presentations. (Note that the PowerPoint files for these presentations are provided on a CD that is attached to the back of this handbook.) As mentioned above, patients should receive a copy of the self-help workbook at the start of the first session. The normal intervention within Level 3 is for patients to attend two sessions facilitated by an audiologist, combined with three sessions facilitated by a psychologist or other mental health provider.

In general, there are several advantages to a group education format (Mensing & Norris, 2003; S. R. Wilson, 1997): (a) Group sessions are both cost-effective and time-efficient. Education and support can be provided to more patients in less time, maximizing available resources; (b) When education is the primary intervention modality, group educational intervention can be equally or more effective than providing the education on an individual basis because of the group-interaction dynamic; (c) Patients often are more motivated to attend group rather than individual sessions because of the encouragement and support that they receive from each other; and (d) Patients who participate in groups tend to form a sense of camaraderie that further motivates them to attend the sessions.

Recent evidence supports the use of group education as a basic form of tinnitus intervention. Group education has been shown to be effective as part of a hierarchical tinnitus management program at a major tinnitus clinic (C. W. Newman & Sandridge, 2005; Sandridge & C. W. Newman, 2005). In addition, we completed a randomized clinical trial (see Chapter 2) evaluating group education for tinnitus in almost 300 patients that showed significantly more reduction in tinnitus severity for patients in the education group as compared to two control groups (J. A. Henry, Loovis, et al., 2007).

PTM group education has been carefully developed to assist patients in directly addressing those life situations when their tinnitus is problematic. The counseling focuses on facilitating self-efficacy and was developed using well-documented principles of patient education and health literacy (J. A. Henry, Zaugg, Myers, Kendall, et al., 2009). PTM counseling thus does not just educate patients *about* tinnitus—it is designed to teach patients *how to self-manage their reactions to tinnitus*. These patients are empowered to make informed decisions about self-management, protecting their ears, and further tinnitus intervention options.

During the first session with the audiologist, the principles of using sound to manage reactions to tinnitus are explained, and participants use the PTM Sound Plan Worksheet (J. A. Henry, Zaugg, Myers, & Kendall, 2009; J. A. Henry et al., 2010a) to develop an individualized "sound plan" to use to manage their most bothersome tinnitus situation. They are instructed to use the sound plan until the next session with the audiologist (approximately two weeks later), at which time they discuss their experiences using the plan and its effectiveness. The audiologist facilitates the discussion and addresses any questions or concerns. Further information about managing reactions to tinnitus is then presented, and the participants revise their sound plan based on the discussion and new information. By the end of the second session with the audiologist, the participants should have learned how to develop, implement, evaluate, and revise a sound plan to manage their most bothersome tinnitus situation. They are encouraged to use the Sound Plan Worksheet on an ongoing basis to write additional sound plans to address other bothersome tinnitus situations. Additional group sessions with the audiologist can be scheduled if needed.

The group education sessions led by a psychologist focus on teaching three cognitive-behavioral therapy (CBT) coping techniques: relaxation, cognitive restructuring ("changing thoughts"), and attention diversion ("planning pleasant activities"). During the first of three sessions with the psychologist, the principles of CBT are explained, and participants use the PTM Changing Thoughts and Feelings Worksheet (J. A. Henry et al., 2010a). The provision of CBT for chronic problems other than tinnitus often involves six to eight sessions (J. L. Henry & P. H. Wilson, 2001). For PTM, only certain components of CBT are taught to minimize the number of group sessions and because other components of CBT, such as education about tinnitus, are provided elsewhere during Level 3 and Level 5.

Patients should have the option of attending additional sessions if further CBT counseling is needed. These additional sessions normally are offered to patients following, and depending on the results of, the Level 4 Interdisciplinary Evaluation. During Level 5 Individualized Support, all CBT modules including psychoeducation, prevention, and planning for relapse and flare-ups are presented in detail according to results of the Level 4 Interdisciplinary Evaluation.

Level 4 Interdisciplinary Evaluation

> **Level 4** involves **in-depth evaluation** of patients who require services beyond Level 3 Group Education.

Patients who are unable to satisfactorily manage their reactions to tinnitus following completion of PTM Levels 2 and 3 require a full evaluation to determine their needs for further intervention. Such an in-depth evaluation is not warranted for the great majority of patients who are able to self-manage reactions to tinnitus with the information and support provided in Levels 2 and 3.

The Level 4 Interdisciplinary Evaluation should include assessments by both an audiologist and a psychologist (or other mental health provider). The audiologist should discuss use of devices and determine if individualized support from an audiologist is warranted. The psychologist's assessment should include screening for psychological conditions that may need to be addressed and a determination if individualized support from a psychologist is warranted. Thus, two appointments normally are required at this level—one with an audiologist and one with a psychologist. Ideally, after both evaluations the audiologist, psychologist, and patient will come to agreement concerning if and how Level 5 intervention should be conducted.

The audiologic tinnitus assessment includes written questionnaires, a structured interview, and, optionally, a psychoacoustic assessment of tinnitus perceptual characteristics. The questionnaires and interview are the key to determining how the tinnitus impacts the patient's life and if individualized support from an audiologist is indicated. Special procedures have been developed for selecting sound-generating devices for tinnitus management using therapeutic sound, including ear-level noise generators and combination instruments, and personal listening devices. The audiology portion of the Level 4 evaluation is used to determine if Level 5 Individualized Support from an audiologist is needed. However, patients who are fitted with ear-level noise generators or combination instruments must progress to Level 5 to ensure proper utilization of the devices.

Screening for symptoms of mental health disorders is considered a requirement at Level 4 if the patient is not already receiving mental health services. Such screenings would include inquiries about depressive and anxious symptomatology, sleep problems, and significant life stressors that may be contributing to one's inability to cope. It is best for the mental health evaluation to be performed by a psychologist or other mental health care provider who is qualified to conduct diagnostic evaluations. If assessment by a mental health care provider is not possible, basic screening for these symptoms can be conducted by any clinician who has been properly trained to use screening tools and who has resources for responding to the outcomes of these screeners. In instances where audiologists (or other nonmental health care providers) are performing screening for referral to mental health, collaborations with primary care are essential to allow for immediate referrals and follow-up as warranted based on mental health screeners. Medical centers and outpatient clinics vary in the types and availability of mental health clinicians. When appropriate mental health care providers are unavailable, collaboration with primary care is necessary to ensure patients receive the best care available at that site.

It should be mentioned that these Level 4 evaluations should take into account patients' impressions about the education they received from the Level 3 classes. It is important to know how useful the information was to patients to focus on building skills that are most likely to provide benefit. Taking this patient-centered approach can help patients feel that they are part of the decision-making process, and increases the likelihood that intervention will be successful.

Level 5 Individualized Support

> **Level 5** is the provision of **one-on-one support** for patients who require longer-term intervention from an audiologist and/or a psychologist.

Level 5 Individualized Support involves repeated appointments with an audiologist and/or a mental health provider (typically a psychologist) who provide one-on-one individualized support to the patient. If ear-level devices are involved in the management program, then appointments with an audiologist are essential to ensure that the devices are working properly and that the patient is using the devices in a manner that is optimal for tinnitus management. Any psychologist providing Level 5 Individualized Support should have experience or adequate training in providing CBT. This foundation is essential to provide effective care.

The audiologic counseling information is essentially the same as what was covered during Level 3 Group Education. However, for Level 5, the audiologist uses a book to facilitate the counseling (*Progressive Tinnitus Management: Counseling Guide*) (J. A. Henry, Zaugg, Myers, & Kendall, 2010b). The book is laid flat on a table between clinician and patient, and works like a flip chart to guide both the audiologist and the patient through the counseling protocol. Patients should attend at least two Level 5 appointments, but they can attend as many as needed. The typical schedule includes appointments at 1, 2, 4, and 6 months following the Level 4 Interdisciplinary Evaluation.

The psychological counseling at Level 5 involves a review of the techniques taught during Level 3 Group Education (and included in the self-help workbook) and an individualized examination of the patient's unique achievements and challenges so far during PTM. Patients learn more about setting and achieving goals via behavioral modification by tracking their progress using clearly defined measures of change. For example, if a patient is having difficulty managing stress, charting stress on a 1-to-10-scale can be effective for quantifying the patient's response to stress and observing change as a result of modifications in behavior. During Level 5, patients learn how to accept their individual strengths and weaknesses while gaining a sense of control in the event that change is realistic and obtainable.

During Level 5 the audiologist and psychologist should collaborate with each other and with the patient to determine what is necessary to provide adequate benefit to the patient. Occasional appointments with both providers may be helpful for clarifying the goals of the interventions and emphasizing a team approach to providing tinnitus care. Options for the patient beyond six months of Level 5 include ongoing psychological symptom management (if warranted), further audiologic intervention (counseling and/or use of ear-level instruments), or other forms of tinnitus intervention that can be provided by an audiologist (tinnitus masking, tinnitus retraining therapy, or neuromonics tinnitus treatment). Some patients may require psychiatric management to address persistent or more serious mental health symptoms that may become evident at any level of PTM. If a psychologist is collaborating then that clinician should make such a referral to psychiatry or the primary care provider.

Conclusion

The five levels of PTM provide a logical, sequential means of working collaboratively with patients to best determine their needs and to provide only the level of care that is needed. It is a basic philosophy of PTM that educating the patient is the most important concern. Thus, patients receive only basic audiology services and self-help education through Level 3. Included in that education is a thorough explanation of the different ways that sound can be used to manage reactions to tinnitus. And, as part of that explanation, patients are taught how sound is used with other sound-based methods of tinnitus management (e.g., tinnitus retraining therapy). Patients should have this understanding before potentially committing to an additional clinical protocol that may be expensive and time-consuming. An important reason why fitting ear-level noise generators or combination instruments is not advocated until Level 4 is that patients need to be fully informed before making such decisions.

Additionally, there continues to be great stigma associated with psychological interventions. Audiologists must be on the frontlines educating patients about the use of psychological interventions for health conditions. Audiologists can help patients with tinnitus feel less concerned about this stigma if they explain the goals of CBT. CBT has been effective in helping patients deal with chronic pain (patients who receive CBT for pain even report decreased levels of pain) (B. M. Hoffman, Papas, Chatkoff, & Kerns, 2007). The analogy between pain and tinnitus is especially useful in introducing the goals of psychological management for tinnitus. Patients should be reassured that clinicians do not think tinnitus is a psychological disorder nor do we think it is "in their heads." It may be important for some patients to hear that clinicians believe their tinnitus is real and very disturbing to them as a validation of their concerns and distress upon introducing the psychologist's role.

If a patient reaches Level 5, then one-on-one support is needed for the patient to better understand the concepts and receive help in trying to learn how to self-manage reactions to tinnitus.

(This is a skill patients likely will need for the rest of their lives so it is important that they fully grasp the concepts.) Furthermore, tinnitus is a dynamic symptom that may change dramatically over the course of the patient's lifetime. If none of the efforts expended through Level 5 works for the patient, then the logical next step is to attempt to modify the procedures, or to try other forms of therapy. As a result of participating in PTM, patients become fully educated about the different uses of sound, and are in a position to make informed decisions about committing to another form of therapy.

PTM is a program that is efficient for audiologists and psychologists and is designed to work in the best interest of patients to help them learn how to self-manage their reactions to tinnitus without getting involved in expensive therapy. If a clinician is committed to one of these other methods, then the framework of PTM can be helpful to more systematically make decisions about the need for a high level of intervention. The interdisciplinary approach of PTM can be modified based on a particular clinic's resources and staffing. Some clinics employ health psychologists or clinical psychologists who specialize in auditory disorders, and who may be especially adept at responding to the psychological needs of patients with tinnitus. Other clinics do not have such clinical resources.

The PTM model is designed for implementation at any clinic that desires to optimize resourcefulness, cost efficiency, and expedience in working with patients who complain of tinnitus. Use of these recommendations should lead to more widespread and consistent tinnitus assessment and intervention by clinicians. Each level of PTM is described in detail in this book.

Case Studies

The following case studies illustrate the PTM approach employed for three patients (Sam, Betty, and Joe). These are somewhat random examples, but they illustrate the range of problems reported by patients and the adaptive nature of PTM to address individual needs.

Case Study: Sam

- **Level 1:** Sam was referred to audiology by primary care for tinnitus and hearing loss complaints.
- **Level 2:** Audiologic evaluation revealed a high frequency sensorineural hearing loss bilaterally. Sam was advised and agreed to be fitted with hearing aids. The brief tinnitus assessment revealed clinically significant tinnitus. Sam's primary care provider and a mental health provider were immediately notified due to his statement "I'm not sure how much I can go on living with this tinnitus."
- **Level 3:** Sam attended group education sessions with the audiologist and psychologist and reported that the education was not enough—he was still very troubled by his tinnitus and wanted more assistance.
- **Level 4:** Sam returned for an interdisciplinary evaluation. The hearing aids were returned for credit and combination instruments were ordered. He and the psychologist agreed that further psychological intervention had potential to be helpful.
- **Level 5:** Sam received individualized ongoing intervention with an audiologist to optimize the use of his combination instruments and to more fully understand the PTM techniques. He met individually with a psychologist to optimize the use of coping techniques based on CBT.

Case Study: Betty

- **Level 1:** Betty was referred to audiology by primary care due to a report of intermittent tinnitus bilaterally.
- **Level 2:** Audiologic evaluation revealed that Betty had normal hearing bilaterally. Assessment of impact of tinnitus revealed that Betty was mildly impacted by her tinnitus. Betty was counseled regarding the test results and her tinnitus. She

was invited to attend Level 3 Group Education.

- **Level 3:** Betty participated in the group education workshops conducted by an audiologist. She obtained the information needed to self-manage her reactions to tinnitus by optimizing her lifestyle and using low level sounds in her environment when the tinnitus was bothersome. She deferred instruction on CBT education or further referral and will contact the clinic if changes or problems are noted.

Case Study: Joe

- **Level 1:** Joe was referred to audiology by his psychologist due to reports that he "dislikes" hearing sound and has very bothersome tinnitus. He stopped socializing last year and avoids all activities that involve moderate levels of sound. The psychologist has been treating him for PTSD.
- **Level 2:** Audiologic evaluation revealed that Joe had moderate hearing loss in his left ear but normal hearing in his right ear. (Referral to otolaryngology and subsequent imaging with MRI indicated no lesions or malformations.) The brief assessment of tinnitus and sound tolerance revealed that Joe was severely impacted by both of these conditions. Because of his severe sound tolerance problem, Joe was advised to participate in the STEM program (see Chapter 6).
- **STEM:** The evaluation determined that Joe's sound tolerance problem involved hyperacusis, misophonia, and phonophobia. Treatment therefore required counseling and support by both an audiologist and a psychologist. In addition, he was fitted with a combination instrument in his left ear and a noise generator in the right ear, and sound was added very gradually via these devices and in his environment. His sound tolerance recovered over a six-month period to the degree that tinnitus became the primary problem. He was advised to attend Level 3 Group Education.
- **Level 3:** Joe participated in all of the group education workshops conducted by both the audiologist and psychologist. Joe learned from the audiologist how to use sound to decrease his awareness of tinnitus and to continue increasing his tolerance to sound. During the CBT workshops he learned the importance of staying active to distract himself from his tinnitus. He became less isolated and began meeting with friends again. The referring psychologist learned about tinnitus from the PTM team and incorporated skills taught during PTM into his PTSD treatment. Joe continues to receive regular follow up from his psychologist. It was decided to not schedule him for a Level 4 Interdisciplinary Evaluation from the audiologist. However, the psychologist and audiologist will consult in approximately 3 months to determine if a Level 4 evaluation is warranted.

4

Level 1 Triage

PTM

Progressive Tinnitus Management

This and the remaining chapters focus on describing detailed procedures for conducting PTM. The present chapter describes procedures for "triaging" patients when they complain of tinnitus at any clinic. Patients report tinnitus to healthcare providers in many different clinics—not just otolaryngology and audiology. Direct points of contact include primary care, psychology, psychiatry, neurology, and oncology. Providers in these (and other) departments may be unaware of clinical resources that are available when patients complain of tinnitus. Guidelines are needed so that clinicians can refer these patients to receive appropriate care.

A guide (Tinnitus Triage Guidelines—Appendix B) has been developed to provide to clinicians as a resource to know how to appropriately refer their patients who complain of tinnitus. The evidence for these guidelines is based on best practices for referring these patients (Harrop-Griffiths et al., 1987; J. A. Henry, Zaugg, et al., 2005a; J. L. Henry & P. H. Wilson, 2001; Wackym & Friedland, 2004). Audiologists see patients in any of PTM Levels 2 to 5, and more comprehensive referral guidelines have been developed for audiologists to use in these levels (J. A. Henry et al., 2008b). Reactions to tinnitus often are best managed using an interdisciplinary approach, thus proper referral and inclusion of a psychologist and otolaryngologist on the "tinnitus team" (when possible) are critical components of PTM.

When a patient complains of tinnitus, the primary concerns are to determine (in order of decreasing priority) if the patient: (a) has a serious medical condition (physical or mental) requiring immediate medical attention; (b) experiences symptoms of a nonurgent medical condition indicating the need for a medical examination; (c) experiences symptoms of a nonurgent psychological condition indicating the need for mental health screening; and (d) has been referred or has none of the symptoms listed above, indicating the current need for an audiologic examination.

Tinnitus Triage Guidelines

The Tinnitus Triage Guidelines (Appendix B) can be used by providers as a quick guide for triaging patients who complain of tinnitus. Following these guidelines should result in appropriate care in most cases. It needs to be emphasized, however, that the guidelines are greatly simplified for clinical expediency. It goes without saying that clinicians must use their clinical judgment to determine the best course of action for each patient. Another caveat is that clinical services for tinnitus are far from being standardized. Clinicians who provide tinnitus services often use very different approaches. Patients who are referred should be advised to become well informed before agreeing to undergo any medical procedure or to enroll in any therapeutic program.

PTM Level 1 Triage shown in the PTM Flowchart (Appendix A) includes a large rectangular text box that lists the basic criteria for referring patients who complain of tinnitus. Depending on the patient's symptoms and other diagnostic factors, there are four possible referrals (as indicated by the four columns in the text box), which are described below. The Tinnitus Triage Guidelines (Appendix B) is an information sheet that can be distributed to providers as a quick guide for triaging their patients who complain about tinnitus. The guidelines can be distributed to clinics that are likely to encounter these patients. The PTM Flowchart (Appendix A) can be printed on the back side of the guidelines (Appendix B) to provide a single sheet with the essential triage/referral information.

Emergency Triage—Urgent Care or Otolaryngology

Idiopathic sudden sensorineural hearing loss (ISSHL) or facial palsy indicates an urgent need to be seen by otolaryngology or urgent care. ISSHL has been defined as hearing loss of at least 20 dB across three adjacent audiometric test frequencies (Battaglia, Burchette, & Cueva, 2008). However, at the time of initial report, patients usually do not have the results of an audiogram. Thus, if the patient reports an unexplained decrease in hearing sensitivity, then ISSHL should be suspected. The loss typically occurs over the course of three days or less and has no clear precipitating cause.

Although the etiology of ISSHL is unknown, possible causes include labyrinthitis (viral or bacterial), vascular disruption, labyrinthine membrane ruptures, immune-mediated mechanisms, abnormal cellular stress responses within the cochlea, and ion transport problems of the stria vascularis (Merchant, Adams, & Nadol, 2005; Trune, 2004). If left untreated, the hearing loss will resolve partially or completely in at least 50% of these patients. This recovery rate may be improved with corticosteroid (glucocorticoid) treatments, particularly if delivered intratympanically (Hamid & Trune, 2008). Although recovery with glucocorticoids often is interpreted as an underlying cochlear inflammation etiology, numerous inner ear ion homeostasis mechanisms also are controlled by corticosteroids (Merchant et al., 2005; Trune, 2004). Thus, conclusions about etiology based on treatment response can be debated, although lack of recovery with glucocorticoids indicates that other treatment options should be pursued.

ISSHL has been referred to as an "otologic emergency" (Goodhill & Harris, 1979). Failure to refer a patient with ISSHL for same-day ENT or urgent care can jeopardize the patient's chances of recovering hearing function. The time course from the onset of symptoms until the initiation of corticosteroid therapy can be a factor in the chances of recovery—the more expediently these patients are seen, the better their prognosis (Jeyakumar, Francis, & Doerr, 2006).

Triage Patient to Mental Health

Some patients require mental health assessment, either because of obvious manifestations of mental health problems or because of expressed suicidal or homicidal ideation. If there is a question about the patient's mental health, then screening tools are available to assist in determining the need for referral (J. A. Henry et al., 2008b). Some patients experience extreme anxiety or depression in reaction to tinnitus and should be referred to a mental health provider the same day symptoms are reported—although this would not be an emergency referral. Suicidal or homicidal ideation warrants special attention, and referral guidelines are available for these patients (G. K. Brown, Henriques, Sosdjan, & Beck, 2004; Hawton, 2001; Kessler, Borges, & Walters, 1999).

In preparation for possible referrals, it is best to establish a relationship with local emergency mental health providers, such as the nearest emergency room, in-house security personnel, or on-call mental health providers. Many sites now have a suicide coordinator. Such mental health providers possess the skills and resources for assessing and responding to a patient's risk of suicide or violence.

Triage Patient to Otolaryngology

Health care providers should refer patients to otolaryngology if certain symptoms coexist with the tinnitus. Patients require a medical examination and a hearing assessment if their symptoms suggest a somatic origin of tinnitus (e.g., pulsatile tinnitus), or if there is ear pain, drainage, or malodor. (Please see Chapters 1 and 5 for information about somatosounds.) Vestibular symptoms also require referral to otolaryngology. The urgency of these referrals is determined by the clinician. Referral to audiology also is indicated in these cases—ideally, patients should see an audiologist first so that audiologic test results are available to the otolaryngologist.

Triage Patient to Audiology

Patients complaining of tinnitus should be referred to audiology if symptoms suggest that a medical examination is not necessary. These patients require a hearing assessment by an audiologist in addition to a brief assessment of the severity of the tinnitus (see Chapter 5) (J. A. Henry et al., 2008b). Triaging patients to audiology requires: (a) symptoms suggest a neurophysiologic (not somatic) origin of tinnitus; (b) no ear pain, drainage, or malodor; (c) no vestibular symptoms; (d) no physical trauma, facial palsy, or ISSHL; and (e) no obvious mental health symptoms or suicidal ideation.

It is important to refer patients to audiologists who have expertise in tinnitus management. These audiologists have the ability to implement several different options for intervention, including use of ear-level devices (hearing aids, "maskers," and combination instruments), educational therapies, and specific sound-based methods of intervention. These audiologists also generally work within a network of providers who specialize in tinnitus. Access to such a network is important to the patient.

It commonly is reported that many patients with tinnitus also suffer from a loudness tolerance problem (usually referred to generically as "hyperacusis"—see Chapter 1 for related definitions). In reality, most patients suspected as "hyperacusic" do not require intervention specific to loudness tolerance. Treatment for the condition generally requires a program of systematic exposure to sound, which is accomplished when implementing sound therapy for tinnitus. For patients with a severe hyperacusis problem, specific therapeutic programs are available (J. A. Henry, Trune, et al., 2007a). Chapter 6 describes the program that is used with PTM for patients who have a severe loudness tolerance problem.

Summary

Patients complain of tinnitus in many different clinics. However, most providers do not know what to tell these patients, nor do they know how to refer them most appropriately. Normally, a referral to audiology is appropriate. However, there are symptoms that suggest urgent or other care is required. We have explained those symptoms and provided the Tinnitus Triage Guidelines (Appendix B), which can be distributed to any clinic that would be the point of contact for patients who complain about tinnitus. These guidelines are appropriate for the majority of patients who complain of tinnitus, but they do not address all patients. It was noted above that the clinician is the final arbiter of any decision to refer a patient.

Different methods for managing reactions to tinnitus can be beneficial to patients when offered by qualified tinnitus specialists. Thus, it is essential to inform patients who complain of tinnitus that good services are available, but that they must be careful to obtain services only from qualified practitioners. Due to the subjective nature of tinnitus, a great many tinnitus "therapies" have been developed that have no scientific basis. Patients bothered by tinnitus have been known to try "just about anything" in an effort to obtain relief. It is unfortunate that this condition is vulnerable to questionable practices. Medical providers of all disciplines thus have the responsibility of providing accurate and positive information to these patients and referring them appropriately for any needed services.

5

Level 2 Audiologic Evaluation

PTM

Progressive Tinnitus Management

Tinnitus is a symptom of dysfunction within the auditory system, and usually is associated with some degree of hearing loss (Axelsson & Ringdahl, 1989; A. Davis & Refaie, 2000; J. L. Henry & P. H. Wilson, 2001; Vernon, 1998). As stated in Chapter 3, an audiologic examination should be the clinical starting point for all patients who complain of tinnitus, unless urgent medical services are required. In addition to the audiology testing, it is critical to determine how much of a patient's complaint is due to a hearing problem and how much is due specifically to the tinnitus. A brief assessment should be performed to determine if intervention specific to tinnitus is warranted.

The objectives of the Level 2 Audiologic Evaluation are to determine the potential need for (a) a medical examination (usually from an otologist or otolaryngologist); (b) mental health screening (from a psychologist, psychiatrist, or other mental health provider); and/or (c) audiologic intervention (which can include intervention for hearing loss, tinnitus, and reduced tolerance to sound) (J. A. Henry et al., 2008b). (Appendix C provides an overview of objectives and procedures of the Level 2 Audiologic Evaluation.)

The Level 2 evaluation includes a standard comprehensive hearing evaluation as well as written questionnaires to assess the patient's perception of the relative impact of hearing and tinnitus problems. Patients who require amplification receive hearing aids, which can result in satisfactory management of reactions to tinnitus with minimal education and support. Any patient who experiences problematic tinnitus (even if they will receive hearing aids) is advised to participate in the Level 3 Group Education workshops.

Tinnitus and Hearing Survey

As discussed in Chapter 3, patients who report problems with tinnitus may really be experiencing problems with hearing. The Tinnitus and Hearing Survey (THS; Appendix D) is a brief questionnaire designed specifically to assist patients and clinicians in determining how much of a patient's reported problem is due to tinnitus and how much is due to hearing problems. The survey also contains two items that screen for sound tolerance problems.

The THS contains three sections. Section A includes four statements that address tinnitus-specific problems unrelated to hearing problems. Section B contains four statements that focus on common hearing problems. The Section B statements are phrased to minimize any perceived effects of tinnitus on hearing function. Higher scores for Section A indicate a tinnitus-specific problem, whereas higher scores for Section B indicate a hearing problem. Results of this survey, along with results of the hearing evaluation, provide the clinician with the information needed to differentiate tinnitus-specific problems from hearing problems. Section C asks patients if they have sound tolerance problems. Affirmative responses to Section C should be discussed with patients to determine the potential need to temporarily suspend the PTM protocol to focus on treating the sound tolerance problem.

After completing the THS, patients should understand that the problems listed in Section A are problems that can be addressed with tinnitus management. Section B problems can be addressed with intervention specific to hearing, regardless of the cause of the hearing problem. Section C addresses possible sound tolerance problems.

Patients who have tinnitus-specific problems should be advised to participate in Level 3 Group Education. Attending the Level 3 workshops will include provision of the self-help workbook (*How to Manage Your Tinnitus: A Step-by-Step Workbook*) (J. A. Henry et al., 2010a). Management options for hearing-related problems include amplification, assistive listening devices, and auditory rehabilitation services. Management options for sound tolerance problems include a special sound tolerance handout (What to Do When Everyday Sounds Are Too Loud—Appendix E), sound desensitization procedures, and participation in the sound tolerance evaluation and management (STEM) protocol (for patients who would have difficulty participating in Level 3 Group Education because of reduced sound tolerance).

PTM Approach to Managing Sound Tolerance Problems

Tinnitus clinicians and researchers often report that a relatively high percentage of patients with tinnitus also suffer from hyperacusis. In reality, many or most patients who are identified as "hyperacusic" do not require intervention specific to sound tolerance. Treatment for reduced sound tolerance usually requires a program of systematic exposure to sound. The PTM sound therapy approach simultaneously addresses reduced sound tolerance. Therefore, sound therapy should be the starting point for PTM patients who have reduced sound tolerance and are able to participate in a program of sound-based tinnitus therapy. The key concern for audiologists is to determine if reduced sound tolerance will interfere with the intervention. Of course, it should be the patient's decision to focus on addressing sound tolerance rather than tinnitus.

Using the Tinnitus and Hearing Survey to Determine Candidacy for Level 3 Group Education

Section A of the THS is used to assist in determining if a patient should attend Level 3 Group Education. Following the steps below can help to ensure that patients do not attend the Level 3 workshops with the misconception that they will learn to manage a hearing-in-noise problem (which patients often believe is the result of the tinnitus blocking sounds they are trying to hear.)

- Explain that group education focuses on finding ways to manage tinnitus-related problems—the workshops do not focus on hearing-related problems.
- Confirm that the patient is interested in attending workshops that address tinnitus-related problems.
- Ensure that the patient understands that participating in Level 3 Group Education does not preclude receiving concurrent services for managing hearing problems.
- Ensure that the patient does not have a sound tolerance problem to such a degree that it would be difficult to participate in the Level 3 workshops.

If the above requirements are met, then the patient likely is a candidate for Level 3 Group Education.

Patient Example: Linda

Using the THS, a patient (Linda) provides a low score for Section A (tinnitus section) and a high score for Section B (hearing section), but reports a severe tinnitus problem. The Level 2 Audiologic Evaluation reveals that Linda has noise induced, high frequency, sensorineural hearing loss. Linda states that the problems listed in Section B are those that she finds most irritating and upsetting, and she believes those problems are caused by the tinnitus. After explaining the objectives of Level 3 Group Education, the audiologist helps her to recognize that she probably would not benefit from a class that focuses on Section A problems. She understands that audiologic management is needed to address the Section B problems. She is happy to receive the self-help workbook (*How to Manage Your Tinnitus: A Step-by-Step Workbook*) to learn more about her tinnitus.

Using the Tinnitus and Hearing Survey to Determine Need for Intervention for Reduced Sound Tolerance

Section C of the THS is used to assist in determining if a patient needs intervention for reduced sound tolerance. Following the steps below can help to ensure that reduced sound tolerance is addressed when needed.

Section C, Item 1

Any patient who reports a sound tolerance problem (of any degree) should receive the sound tolerance handout (What to Do When Everyday Sounds Are Too Loud—Appendix E).

Section C, Item 2

If a patient reports that a sound tolerance problem would make it difficult to attend the Level 3 workshops, this should be thoroughly discussed to ascertain that the patient would indeed have difficulty attending a group workshop specifically because of a sound tolerance problem (and not because of some other reason such as social anxiety, transportation problems, severe hearing loss, etc.). If sound tolerance is such a problem that the patient cannot continue with the normal PTM protocol, then a separate protocol should be undertaken to address the sound tolerance problem. The STEM protocol (Chapter 6) was developed for this purpose. Once the sound tolerance problem is sufficiently resolved, then the patient can re-enter the PTM protocol if necessary to address any tinnitus problems. Normally, reentry into PTM would involve the patient attending the Level 3 workshops (see Appendix A).

Tinnitus Handicap Inventory

Standardized tinnitus questionnaires are used to obtain a global index score of a patient's perceived tinnitus severity, and many questionnaires are available for this purpose (C. W. Newman & Sandridge, 2004). A tinnitus-severity index score from a tinnitus questionnaire, however, should not be relied on as the sole indicator of the degree to which tinnitus affects a patient's life (as explained in the next section).

A tinnitus questionnaire provides a standardized baseline of the patient's perceived problem due to tinnitus, and it is essential to acquire this baseline prior to any testing or counseling. We recommend using the Tinnitus Handicap Inventory (THI—Appendix F) (C. W. Newman et al., 1996) for this purpose because it is one of the most widely used and best documented of the tinnitus questionnaires that currently are available. For management with PTM, the THI can serve as the primary outcome instrument. Patients should complete the THI to assess outcomes at intervals (e.g., every 3 months) during ongoing intervention, and prior to terminating intervention.

The THI contains 25 statements, and response choices are "no" (0 points), "sometimes" (2 points), and "yes" (4 points). The index score ranges from 0 to 100. Handicap severity can be categorized based on the THI index score as follows (Handscomb, 2006):

- Severe (58–100)
- Moderate (38–56)
- Mild (18–36)
- No handicap (0–16)

A change in the total index score of at least 20 points has been reported to indicate a statistically and clinically significant change in self-perceived tinnitus handicap (C. W. Newman & Sandridge, 2004).

A 10-question screening version of the THI (THI-S—see Appendix F) also can be used (C. W. Newman, Sandridge, & Bolek, 2008). The THI-S includes 10 of the same questions as the full-length THI and usually takes less than two minutes to complete. Comparison of the THI-S to the THI revealed a high correlation ($r = 0.90$). An index score of at least 6 points (out of a possible 40 points) on the THI-S was established as a fence for recommending follow-up. A change of more than 10 points is considered a significant clinical difference.

How Do the Tinnitus Handicap Inventory and Tinnitus and Hearing Survey Differ?

The THI and THS are used to accomplish different objectives, and each is important for PTM.

The THI is a statistically validated and widely recognized tool for assessing self-perceived tinnitus handicap, making it appropriate for standardized assessment of outcomes of clinical intervention. A patient's index score from any tinnitus questionnaire, including the THI, is vulnerable to influence from hearing problems and cannot be relied on as the sole indicator of candidacy for Level 3 Group Education.

The THS is not a validated outcome instrument, and therefore should not be used as a primary measure of outcome of intervention. The THS was designed to differentiate tinnitus-specific versus hearing-specific problems, which is helpful for determining if a patient should attend Level 3 Group Education. The THS can be used informally to monitor relative progress alleviating tinnitus problems versus hearing problems.

Hearing Handicap Inventory

The Hearing Handicap Inventory (HHI) is a self-administered questionnaire that assesses self-perceived handicap imposed by hearing loss. Use of the HHI is recommended as a standard assessment tool for all patients undergoing Level 2 Audiologic Evaluation. Results of the HHI provide additional information to better understand how much of a patient's complaints about tinnitus may be attributable to hearing handicap, which contributes to a more accurate interpretation of patients' responses to the THI and THS.

Four versions of the HHI can be used. The Hearing Handicap Inventory for the Elderly (HHIE) is intended for patients age 65 and older (Ventry & Weinstein, 1982). The Hearing Handicap Inventory for Adults (HHIA) is intended for patients less than 65 years of age (C. W. Newman, Weinstein, Jacobson, & Hug, 1990). Both the HHIE and HHIA are 25-item self-assessment scales that include two subscales (emotional and social/situational). The HHIA differs from the HHIE only in that it includes questions about occupational effects of hearing loss. The screening versions of the HHIE (HHIE-S) and the HHIA (HHIA-S) each include 10 items and can be completed in 5 minutes or less (Lichtenstein, Bess, Logan, & Burger, 1990; Ventry & Weinstein, 1983). The HHIE-S can be used with all patients and is recommended for routine use at the Level 2 Audiologic Evaluation (Appendix G).

Assessment of Auditory Function

A standard audiologic evaluation provides the information necessary to determine need for referral for medical evaluation and to determine candidacy for audiologic hearing intervention. This is routine practice for audiologists, but some of the procedures warrant special considerations when patients present with tinnitus.

Otoscopy is performed routinely prior to placing earphones for audiometric testing. Even a small amount of cerumen on the tympanic membrane can create a mass effect resulting in a high frequency conductive hearing loss and tinnitus (Schechter & J. A. Henry, 2002). Therefore, it is important to consider this possibility when performing otoscopy.

Pulsed tones often are recommended for use when evaluating pure-tone thresholds in patients with tinnitus (Douek & Reid, 1968; Fulton & Lloyd, 1975; Green, 1972; Yantis, 1994). Investigations, however, have revealed that hearing thresholds generally are the same whether tones are presented in the pulsed or continuous mode (J. A. Henry & Meikle, 1999; Hochberg & Waltzman, 1972; Mineau & Schlauch, 1997). It is acceptable to use either pulsed or continuous tones for threshold testing, although the use of pulsed tones may assist some patients in distinguishing between the tones and the tinnitus, especially when the tinnitus pitch is close to the test frequency.

Some patients with tinnitus have trouble tolerating louder sounds, and some report that loud sounds make their tinnitus louder. It is important to use caution when conducting suprathreshold audiometric testing. The following guidelines can be helpful:

- Use the softest effective masking sounds during traditional audiometry (the need for masking can be reduced by using insert earphones that increase interaural attenuation).
- Use conservative levels of sound during word recognition testing.
- Approach reflex threshold and decay testing with particular caution as some patients have trouble tolerating the sounds used in these tests. In no instance should pure tones be delivered above 105 dB HL. Speech stimuli should not be delivered above 100 dB HL.

Assessment of Potential Need for Otolaryngology Exam

As the ideal, every patient complaining of tinnitus would be examined by an otolaryngologist or otologist (Perry & Gantz, 2000). However, this may not be practical or realistic in some settings. Audiologists sometimes are the only health care providers who evaluate patients with tinnitus complaints. Audiologists must be aware of symptoms and conditions that indicate the need for referral to otolaryngology, which include:

- Symptoms consistent with vestibular schwannoma or other retrocochlear pathology
- Symptoms consistent with Ménière's disease
- Symptoms consistent with somatic origin (i.e., vascular, muscular, skeletal, respiratory, or TMJ) of tinnitus (see next section below)
- Ear pain, drainage, or malodor
- Vestibular symptoms
- New-onset tinnitus or hearing loss
- Progressive tinnitus (tinnitus that is perceived as changing in loudness, pitch, and/or timbre over time)
- Significant conductive loss of undetermined etiology
- Unilateral or grossly asymmetric hearing loss.

The most common type of tinnitus is associated with noise-induced hearing loss. These patients usually report that their tinnitus has been fairly stable for years. This common form of tinnitus cannot be corrected surgically, nor is it life threatening. Although a medical exam always is in the patient's best interest, an otologic exam may be eliminated if *all* of the following conditions apply:

- All symptoms and conditions that indicate the need for referral to otolaryngology (listed above) have been ruled out.
- Patient reports a history of noise exposure and concurrent or subsequent onset of tinnitus.
- Tinnitus is symmetric and nonpulsatile.
- Audiogram is consistent with a diagnosis of symmetric sensorineural hearing loss.

Symptoms of Somatosounds

We briefly described somatic tinnitus (somatosounds) in Chapter 1. It is important for clinicians to realize that many sounds of the head and neck are normal (Hazell, 2003). When we swallow we hear a clicking sound. There is a great deal of blood pulsing through the head and neck at any given time—causing constant loud pulsations (that we normally don't perceive). The carotid artery passes within about 6mm of the cochlea, and we occasionally can hear sounds of the heart through this artery. Additional sounds are caused by joints and muscles, the eustachian tube, and air passing through the airways. Although all of these sounds are considered normal, they become abnormal when heard on a daily basis or when they cause distress.

Somatosounds generally can be categorized as pulsatile and nonpulsatile (Hazell, 1998b). Pulsatile somatounds include venous hums, vascular loops, and carotid transmissions. Venous hums are caused by turbulent blood flow through the jugular bulb, which is a protrusion into the mastoid cavity (close to the middle ear) of the internal jugular vein. A large amount of blood flows rapidly through the jugular vein, causing vibration of the vein walls that is perceived as a humming noise. This is easily evaluated by an otolaryngologist and is a benign condition. Vascular loops within the internal auditory canal can compress the auditory nerve (Nuttall et al., 2004). This compression can cause auditory nerve activity that may be perceived as sound, which may be pulsatile (Møller, 1995; Nuttall et al., 2004). Surgery can remediate tinnitus caused by vascular compression of the auditory nerve. Carotid transmissions refers to any transmission of sound to the cochlea from the carotid artery. This often is caused by stenosis of the carotid artery, but also can include transmission of heart murmurs (Hazell, 1998b; Lockwood et al., 2004).

There are many other potential causes of pulsatile tinnitus, which have been described (Lockwood et al., 2004; Sismanis, 1998, 2003, 2007). Although rare, life-threatening pathology may be associated with pulsatile tinnitus (Sismanis, 2007). It thus is critical to establish an appropriate diagnosis for these patients. In general, a patient with pulsatile tinnitus should be medically evaluated to rule out potential vascular or neurologic conditions that require medical or surgical treatment. These may include hypertension, hyperthyroidism, carotid blockage, glomus tumor, arteriovenous malformation, aneurisms, and so forth. Glomus tumors are rare, but they are the most common tumor of the middle ear and second most common of the temporal bone (second to vestibular schwannoma) (Moffat & Hardy, 1989). Any mention of tumors to patients can cause alarm and anxiety. It therefore is important to assure patients that these tumors are rare, and if they occur they usually are benign.

Nonpulsatile somatosounds include patulous eustachian tube, palatal myoclonus, and tensor tympani syndrome (Hazell, 1998b). A patulous eustachian tube remains open abnormally. This condition often is misdiagnosed as a blocked eustachian tube (Schuknecht, 1993). Symptoms can include a sense of ear fullness, respiratory noises, and autophony (abnormal loudness of one's own voice). Palatonal myoclonus is caused by rapid contractions of the soft palate musculature (Hazell, 1998b; Lockwood et al., 2004). These contractions may be associated with contractions of other muscles in the head and neck. The contractions can cause the eustachian tube to open and close, giving the perception of an irregular clicking/snapping sound in one or both ears. Tensor tympani syndrome is caused by spasms of the tensor tympani muscle that produces a fluttering low frequency sound (Hazell, 1998b). The sound may be correlated with the sensation of an insect fluttering in the ear canal. This condition generally is benign but may be alleviated by sectioning of the tensor tympani muscle.

Somatically Modulated Tinnitus

Some patients report that movements or manipulations of the eyes, head, neck, jaw, or shoulder can cause changes in the loudness or pitch of their tinnitus. This phenomenon is referred to as "somatically modulated tinnitus." It has been reported by some investigators that the phenomenon is much more prevalent than previously thought—with up to 80% of patients reporting that their tinnitus can be modulated somatically when asked the right questions (Levine, 2004). If a patient does report that movement of the head or neck can change the loudness or pitch of the tinnitus, then the question arises as to how to properly refer these patients. In general, all of these patients should be evaluated by an audiologist. The audiologist then can determine if a referral to otolaryngology or neurology is necessary.

Administer Tinnitus Problem Checklist (optional procedure)

To conclude the Level 2 Audiologic Evaluation, it is important to review results of the Tinnitus and Hearing Survey, Tinnitus Handicap Inventory, Hearing Handicap Inventory, and hearing assessment.

The patient should understand that problems listed in Section A of the Tinnitus and Hearing Survey are specific to tinnitus and are addressed in Level 3 Group Education, and that problems in Section B are addressed by an audiologist and are not covered in Level 3 Group Education.

If the patient has a tinnitus-specific problem, and if time permits, then the Tinnitus Problem Checklist (Appendix H) can be helpful. Use of the checklist is the starting point for teaching a patient how to use sound to manage tinnitus, as described in the self-help workbook (*How to Manage Your Tinnitus: A Step-by-Step Workbook*) (J. A. Henry et al., 2010a). Using the checklist provides structure to talk to patients about any problems they experience that are caused by the tinnitus. The checklist also gives the patient information that is useful to understanding how the workbook can be used, which is an advantage to patients who receive a copy of the workbook.

Hearing Aid Evaluation (if warranted)

Most patients with tinnitus have some degree of hearing loss and hearing aids sometimes can adequately ameliorate both their hearing and tinnitus problems (Surr et al., 1999, 1985). All patients should be advised of the potential for hearing aids to alleviate tinnitus as a secondary benefit. In some instances, hearing aids can be used primarily for managing tinnitus with improved hearing as a secondary benefit (J. A. Henry et al., 2008b; J. A. Henry, Zaugg, et al., 2005a; Searchfield, 2005).

The Flowchart for Assessment and Fitting of Ear-Level Instruments (Appendix I) shows the clinical actions for PTM Levels 2 through 5—with the focus on ear-level instruments. The Level 2 Audiologic Evaluation includes an assessment of candidacy for hearing aids. If the patient is a hearing aid candidate, then hearing aids are fitted as appropriate. The preferred approach to providing patients with ear-level instruments is to dispense only hearing aids at Level 2 and not to provide ear-level combination instruments or noise/sound generators until after patients have completed Level 3 Group Education. Noise generators and combination instruments should not be an option for patients until they have learned about and implemented different strategies of using sound for tinnitus management as addressed in Level 3 Group Education. The knowledge and experience of using sound to manage tinnitus gained during Level 3 allows patients to make informed decisions about using noise generators and combination instruments. Many patients can learn how to self-manage their tinnitus without having to use special ear-level instruments. If instrument use is warranted, then the proper use of these devices requires multiple appointments with an audiologist who understands their use within the context of PTM.

Although we generally recommend fitting only hearing aids at Level 2, recent developments need to be considered. In the past, combination instruments included amplification features that were limited relative to hearing aids. Patients who were fitted with combination instruments often did not receive amplification that optimally addressed their hearing loss. That situation has changed with the recent introduction of new combination instruments from a number of hearing aid companies. These combination instruments do not sacrifice hearing aid features so patients can be fitted with these devices as high-quality hearing aids. When fitting such combination instruments at Level 2, it might be preferable to not use the noise feature of the devices until the patient has attended a Level 3 workshop—to ensure that the patient fully understands the different uses of therapeutic sound before actually using it with these devices.

Patients with Hearing Loss

At Level 2, patients with hearing loss are provided amplification, assistive listening devices, and education in communication strategies as necessary to maximize their hearing function. Since impaired hearing may be the patient's primary problem (often unknowingly prior to the hearing evaluation), it is essential to optimize hearing function. Furthermore, patients who progress to Level 3 Group Education require adequate hearing in order for them to comprehend the presentation and group discussion. Patients who receive hearing aids and/or assistive listening devices will receive instruction in how to use these devices (along with many other uses of sound and sound devices) for the management of tinnitus.

Patients With Normal Hearing

For Level 2 patients who have normal hearing and problematic tinnitus, Level 3 Group Education is recommended. In the group workshop, these patients learn how to use sound (from many sources) to manage their reactions to tinnitus. Some of these patients will acquire the skills needed for satisfactory management and will not need further intervention. Others may require further help after completing Level 3, at which point they should be considered for a Level 4 Interdisciplinary Evaluation that normally includes an evaluation for ear-level noise generators. Because of their personal experience using sound to manage tinnitus at Level 3, these patients should be well prepared to participate fully in any decision about using ear-level noise generators.

Use of Hearing Aids With PTM

For audiologists, the provision of hearing aids is a routine service with an established skill set. Audiologists are trained and experienced in the selection and fitting of hearing aids for the purpose of improving hearing. If hearing aids are incorporated into management for tinnitus, then the audiologist essentially has the training necessary to perform this service (J. A. Henry, Zaugg, et al., 2005a). The method of PTM makes full use of these existing skills to apply them directly to addressing tinnitus. There are, however, special considerations for the use of hearing aids with these patients (Appendix J).

Hearing Aids for Managing Reactions to Tinnitus

Special considerations are important with respect to using hearing aids for tinnitus management (these points are summarized briefly in Appendix J):

- The ear canal should be left open as much as possible (or venting should be maximal—as appropriate for slope and degree of loss) to allow normal entry of environmental sound (especially lowest frequency sounds that are not amplified by the hearing aids) and to reduce the sensation of occlusion. Both factors can contribute to reducing tinnitus perception.
- Hearing aids with feedback reduction circuitry can facilitate the use of open-ear design hearing aids, or larger vent diameters.
- Special noise suppression circuitry actually can be a detriment to patients with tinnitus, as noise suppression could eliminate some background sound that might be helpful for these patients. What may be a goal for optimal hearing aid performance may be at cross-purposes for tinnitus management. If a patient with tinnitus has hearing aids with multiple memories, then a consideration is to program one of the memories to minimize noise reduction (as the "tinnitus" setting) with the microphone set to omnidirectional, and adjusted to minimize the reduction of background sound. Some hearing aids offer "music" settings, or other settings that minimize use of algorithms to eliminate nonspeech sounds.
- Some hearing aids offer sound generator settings that can be activated/reprogrammed after Level 3 Group Education is provided if amplification alone does not ameloriate effects of tinnitus.
- Reduced levels of internal noise also can be detrimental to tinnitus management. In older hearing aids, the floor noise of hearing aids often was helpful for tinnitus patients.

Benefits of Amplification for Patients With Tinnitus

Beneficial effects on tinnitus from the use of amplification may be due to:

- Amelioration of communicative difficulties caused by hearing loss but attributed to tinnitus

- Alleviation of stress associated with difficult listening situations
- Increase in ambient sound that can reduce the effects of tinnitus (typically, ambient sound makes tinnitus less noticeable)
- Stimulation of impaired portions of the auditory system that often are deprived of sound.

Refer for Mental Health Screening (if indicated)

Certain mental health disorders are known to be associated with the presence and severity of tinnitus. Clinical depression and anxiety often affect patients who experience the most problematic tinnitus (Dobie, 2003; Halford & Anderson, 1991; Kirsch et al., 1989). In addition, some patients suffer from post-traumatic stress disorder (PTSD). PTSD is suspected if the patient reports having been exposed to a trauma and subsequently experienced nightmares, flashbacks, exaggerated startle responses, or excessive anxiety or fear. The traumatic event does not need to be recent for a patient to experience PTSD.

Although depression, anxiety, and PTSD commonly are associated with tinnitus, many other mental health disorders also may present along with tinnitus. These can include substance abuse (opiates, amphetamines, sedatives, cocaine, marijuana, hallucinogens, alcohol, etc.), bipolar disorder, psychotic disorders, attention-deficit/hyperactivity disorder, panic, phobias, and obsessive-compulsive disorder (J. A. Henry et al., 2008b). All of these conditions, and others, present in clinical settings in varying degrees. It is important to not limit screening and referral to only mental health conditions that have known or suspected interactions with tinnitus. Failure to refer patients for possible mental health conditions reduces the likelihood of achieving the desired outcomes from any tinnitus intervention. The concern for so many potential mental health disorders in patients with tinnitus can present a conundrum for audiologists, which speaks to the need for a psychologist to be on the "tinnitus team."

If indicated by a patient's comments or behavior during the Level 2 evaluation, screening for mental health issues should be performed (unless the patient already is diagnosed with a mental health condition[s] and currently is receiving care accordingly). Mental health screening also can be done at any stage of PTM at the clinician's discretion. If possible, such screening ideally is conducted by a mental health or primary care provider. In most medical centers, primary care offers competent and efficient mental health screening services. Thus, it usually is preferable to refer patients who are suspected of mental health conditions to primary care for screening. However, different facilities may handle mental health screening differently so it is important to determine the procedures used at each facility. If screening is not available elsewhere, it can be useful for an audiologist to use specific questionnaires to screen for the more common comorbid conditions of sleep problems, PTSD, anxiety problems, and symptoms of depression (see Chapter 8).

Refer for Assessment of Sleep Disorder (if indicated)

Sleep disorders are the most common problem reported by patients who are bothered by tinnitus (Axelsson & Ringdahl, 1989; Jakes et al., 1985; Meikle et al., 2004; Tyler & Baker, 1983). Patients with sleep disorders also tend to report the most severe tinnitus (Erlandsson, Hallberg, & Axelsson, 1992; Folmer & Griest, 2000; Meikle, Vernon, & Johnson, 1984; Scott, Lindberg, Melin, & Lyttkens, 1990). These patients may need specialized treatment from a physician, mental health professional, and/or sleep disorders clinician.

It is important to question a patient about details of a reported sleep disorder to determine if referral is needed. In some cases a sleep disorder can be related to a serious medical condition. It also is important to distinguish between insomnia and sleep apnea. Insomnia is a problem with initiating or maintaining sleep, which typically does not have serious medical effects. Sleep apnea is a condition whereby breathing during sleep is disrupted and can have serious health effects such as stroke. Patients who report snoring, morning headaches, gasping or choking upon waking, or those who have a bed partner who reports the presence of these indications of sleep apnea, should be referred to primary care for assessment.

Managing Sleep Disorder

If a patient's sleep disorder is a direct consequence of the tinnitus, then effective tinnitus management may resolve the sleep problem. This requires the appropriate use of sound in the sleep environment. In most cases, this should be attempted prior to referring the patient out for insomnia treatment. The use of sound is harmless and inexpensive, whereas insomnia treatment can involve medications, side effects, and significant costs. Strategies for improving sleep when tinnitus is a problem are explained in the Level 3 workshops, and are included in the self-help workbook (J. A. Henry et al., 2010a).

Prescription Drugs and Tinnitus

No prescription drug has been developed specifically for tinnitus. However, some antidepressant or anxiolitic medications such as amitryptiline or lorazepam may reduce symptoms. These drugs most commonly are used to address coexisting sleep disorders and mental health disorders—primarily depression and anxiety (Dobie, 2004a; J. A. Henry, Zaugg, et al., 2005a; Robinson, Viirre, & Stein, 2004). These studies conclude that medical management of sleep and mental health problems can be a helpful component of an overall approach to managing reactions to tinnitus.

Certain medications can trigger or exacerbate tinnitus, including aspirin, NSAIDS, loop diuretics, and quinine. Normally, fairly high doses are required to cause tinnitus effects, and the effects usually are temporary. Drugs used to treat mental health and sleep conditions also may trigger or exacerbate tinnitus. Patients have reported exacerbation of tinnitus due to alcohol and caffeine. Ototoxicity from aminoglycosides and platinum-containing chemotherapeutic drugs are well-known causes of hearing loss and tinnitus, and these effects often are irreversible (Fausti et al., 1995; Rachel et al., 2002).

The only way to know if a medication alleviates tinnitus is through trial-and-error (e.g., some antidepressants can cause or exacerbate tinnitus as a side effect). This generally is what is done by physicians who attempt to use medications to treat tinnitus. It is better for patients if they can be helped with counseling and the proper use of sound rather than receiving medications that can have harmful side effects or result in dependency/addiction.

Self-Help Workbook

The self-help workbook (*How to Manage Your Tinnitus: A Step-by-Step Workbook*) (J. A. Henry et al., 2010a) can be given to patients either at the end of the Level 2 Audiologic Evaluation, or at the beginning of Level 3 Group Education. It generally is preferable to withhold provision of the workbook until the patient shows up for the first Level 3 workshop—for a number of reasons: (a) Anticipating receiving the workbook increases the likelihood that patients will participate in Level 3. Attending the workshops increases the likelihood that patients will learn and benefit from the self-help information. Also, increasing the group size can improve the likelihood of meaningful interactions amongst group members. (b) Many patients believe that reducing the loudness of their tinnitus is the only way to feel better and may be disillusioned by the workbook since it does not offer that option. These patients may not even attempt to implement the ideas contained in the workbook and thus may only be able to benefit from the workbook if guided through it by a clinician (and in a group setting sometimes it may be other group members who are best able to influence a patient that the ideas in the workbook can be helpful). (c) Providing the workbook as a patient is leaving the clinic decreases the likelihood that the patient and clinician will discuss the concepts. Discussion fosters interest and learning, and is more likely to lead to the patient making behavioral changes that will reduce reactions to tinnitus and increase quality of life.

We recommend offering to provide patients with their own copy of the workbook when they come to the first Level 3 workshop. Patients also should be told about the 13-minute tinnitus video that they can view online (http://www.ncrar.research.va.gov/ForVets/Tinnitus.asx). This video was professionally produced by VA Employee Education System and provides basic information that can help to increase interest in learning the concepts that are taught in the workbook and Level 3 workshops. The DVD with the 13-minute video is available from the NCRAR (or from any of the authors of this handbook) and can be used in the clinic to show to patients. Most patients find the video to be entertaining and informative.

Summary

The great majority of patients who report tinnitus also have some degree of hearing loss. The essential first step in providing clinical services for these patients normally is to assess their hearing function. Using the triage guidelines described in the previous chapter, these patients may require a medical and/or a mental health examination. At a minimum, however, all patients who report tinnitus should be assessed by an audiologist who can determine what services are needed, including: (a) medical exam; (b) mental health screening; and (c) audiologic intervention for hearing loss, tinnitus, and/or hyperacusis.

The Level 2 Audiologic Evaluation consists mainly of a conventional audiologic assessment. Because the patient reports tinnitus, a brief assessment of tinnitus impact is performed. The primary tool for assessing tinnitus impact is the Tinnitus and Hearing Survey (THS). Results of the THS should be discussed with the patient to determine if tinnitus-specific intervention is appropriate. In addition to the THS, it is recommended to administer the Tinnitus Handicap Inventory (THI) and Hearing Handicap Inventory for the Elderly—screening version (HHIE-S). Results of the THI serve as a statistically validated baseline for assessing outcomes of the tinnitus intervention. Results of the HHIE-S facilitate interpretation of the THS and THI, and serve as a statistically validated baseline for assessing outcomes of clinical services specific to hearing loss. Combined, these three questionnaires provide useful data for documenting a patient's complaints and for determining clinical services that may be needed.

6

Sound Tolerance Evaluation and Management (STEM)

PTM

Progressive Tinnitus Management

As described in the previous chapter, the Tinnitus and Hearing Survey (Appendix D) includes two items in Section C that screen for reduced sound tolerance. The first item determines if a patient perceives that he or she has a loudness tolerance problem, and, if so, how much of a problem. If a problem is reported, then the second item is used to determine if the patient would experience difficulty attending the Level 3 workshops due to the sound/loudness tolerance problem. If the patient reports a sound tolerance problem, but can attend the workshops to address a tinnitus problem, then the patient normally should attend the group sessions. Some patients, however, may express a strong desire to focus on their sound tolerance problem rather than the tinnitus, and those wishes should be honored even if the patient is capable of participating in the Level 3 workshops.

During the Level 3 workshops, patients learn how to use therapeutic sound in various ways for managing reactions to tinnitus. All of the suggestions for using sound to manage tinnitus also are relevant for managing a sound tolerance problem. That is, if the patient follows the suggestions for using therapeutic sound, then not only can the sound help with the tinnitus, but it also can help to increase tolerance to sound (Formby, Sherlock, & Gold, 2002). If the patient indicates on the second item of Section C that he or she would not be comfortable attending Level 3 Group Education, then that should alert the clinician to discuss sound tolerance with the patient and consider scheduling a special appointment to evaluate the sound tolerance problem. As mentioned above, some patients may just wish to focus on their sound tolerance problem.

What Is STEM?

The sound tolerance evaluation and management (STEM) protocol is an adjunct program primarily for patients who have a sound tolerance problem that precludes them from participating in the PTM protocol. These patients are identified at the Level 2 Audiologic Evaluation as requiring the special STEM program (see Chapter 5). Their progress through PTM is suspended temporarily until they complete the STEM program. Sound-based intervention that patients receive through the STEM program also may resolve their tinnitus problem, in which case they may not need to resume the PTM program (see PTM Flowchart—Appendix A). As a general rule, however, any patients with problems specific to tinnitus should be advised to participate in Level 3 Group Education.

The STEM evaluation appointment can include three components: administering the Sound Tolerance Interview (STI), testing loudness discomfort levels (LDLs), and trial use of ear-level instruments. Only the STI is essential for the evaluation, that is, it is essential to conduct an in-depth interview to fully understand the nature and severity of the problem, and to develop an appropriate management plan. The STI also provides data that can be used as a baseline to evaluate progress over time.

All patients who participate in STEM should receive counseling for reduced sound tolerance. A counseling protocol is provided in the patient counseling book (*Progressive Tinnitus Management: Counseling Guide*) (J. A. Henry et al., 2010b).

Sound Tolerance Interview

The six-question Sound Tolerance Interview (STI) (Appendix K) fits within the framework of PTM and serves to guide the STEM evaluation procedures. The interview starts with a series of questions (embedded in Question 1) to determine if the use of hearing aids contributes to the patient's reported sound tolerance problem. Questions 2 through 5 are used to obtain details concerning the kinds of sounds and activities that are problematic, and the degree of the problem in each case. Question 6 is intended to determine if the patient overprotects his or her ears through the use of hearing protection. (Overuse of hearing protection can sustain or exacerbate a sound tolerance problem.)

Treatment for Reduced Sound Tolerance

As explained in the patient handout "What to Do When Everyday Sounds Are Too Loud" (Appendix E), the essence of treatment for a sound tolerance problem is the systematic use of sound to decrease sensitivity to sound. Although there are different manifestations of a sound tolerance problem (as described in Chapter 1), a generic approach to treatment usually is adequate. The treatment involves increasing ambient levels of sound (with the possible use of ear-level instruments) as well as increasing activities involving active listening to sounds that the patient finds enjoyable. This combined approach thus includes: (a) passive listening procedures, which address general hypersensitivity to sound, and (b) active listening procedures, which address the emotional components of a sound tolerance problem. Procedures for addressing these different components individually are available using the method of tinnitus retraining therapy (TRT) (J. A. Henry, Trune, Robb, & P. J. Jastreboff, 2007a, 2007b; P. J. Jastreboff & Hazell, 2004). These TRT procedures can be used if the clinician has familiarity with the procedures.

Counseling for reduced sound tolerance is provided in a structured format using the patient counseling book (*Progressive Tinnitus Management: Counseling Guide*) (J. A. Henry et al., 2010b), which contains a special section for this purpose. The counseling book functions like a flip chart to facilitate the one-on-one counseling. The content of the counseling corresponds closely with the patient handout "What to Do When Everyday Sounds Are Too Loud" (Appendix E). The handout normally is provided to patients at the Level 2 Audiologic Evaluation if they report any degree of a sound tolerance problem. The counseling leads to an explanation of the Sound Tolerance Worksheet (Appendix L). Patients learn how to complete this special worksheet to develop customized plans for self-managing their sound tolerance problem using therapeutic sound.

Testing Loudness Discomfort Levels (optional procedure)

Testing loudness discomfort levels (LDLs) is less important than information obtained from the Sound Tolerance Interview. At the audiologist's discretion, LDLs can be tested for patients who go through the STEM program, but LDL testing is not normally recommended. Although this is a debatable point, we consider LDL testing to be nonessential even when a patient has a severe problem with reduced sound tolerance because: (a) testing LDLs can cause discomfort and anxiety in patients; (b) the validity of LDLs as a measure of loudness tolerance in daily life has not been established; and (c) the results of LDL testing do not normally guide intervention procedures.

If a patient has reduced tolerance to sound, it is our position that the best indicator for establishing the degree of a sound tolerance problem, and to monitor progress during treatment, is the patient's subjective report—which is facilitated through administration of a structured interview with the STI (see Appendix K). Results of the interview define the problem and indicate the course of action that should be taken, regardless of the results of LDL testing. Some audiologists choose to do LDL testing, which is acceptable as long as the patient is comfortable with the procedures. LDL procedures are described further below.

Definition of LDL

The threshold level of discomfort for a sound defines that sound's LDL. The LDL should reflect the level just below physical discomfort and not just fear that the sound is going to become too loud (a common manifestation of phonophobia). Clinical LDL testing can be done using pure tones, speech stimuli, and narrow and broadband noise. Using pure tones, LDLs can be obtained at various audiometric frequencies, establishing the upper limit of the auditory dynamic range for each frequency tested. Sounds would be tolerated comfortably anywhere within the dynamic range.

Measuring Tonal LDLs

(Please refer to *Loudness Discomfort Levels—Clinical Guide*—Appendix M.) If tonal LDLs are tested, then they should be obtained minimally at octave frequencies between 1 and 8 kHz. LDL testing may be performed at additional frequencies and with other types of auditory stimuli. Patients often are inconsistent when providing repeated LDLs within a test session. Some providers therefore measure each LDL twice. This is done by first obtaining the LDLs in each ear, then repeating the entire set of measurements.

Instructions to Patients

Loudness discomfort levels can vary considerably depending on the test instructions given to the patient, and on the patient's interpretation of the instructions. It is essential to read standardized scripted instructions verbatim and to ask patients to repeat back the task as they understand it. Patients are instructed, *"You will listen to different tones. Each tone will be made slightly louder in steps. Tell me when the loudness of the tone would be ok for 3 seconds, but would not be OK for more than 3 seconds."* The objective is to identify the level for each frequency at which any further increase would cause discomfort.

Audiometric Procedures

Testing in each ear should start at 1000 Hz, with successive frequencies ordered from lowest to highest. The first tone is presented at the approximate most comfortable level (usually 60 dB HL is appropriate to start). Each tone is presented for 1 to 2 seconds, and successive tones are raised in 5 dB steps until the LDL is reported. At each new frequency, the starting level should be about 20 dB below the previous frequency's LDL.

As LDL testing is probably the patient's least favorite procedure, it is important to perform the testing as rapidly as possible (without compromising the measures). If two sets of measures are obtained, only the second set should be reported. Reliability of responding also should be noted.

In-Clinic Trial Use of Ear-Level Instruments (optional procedure)

After the sound tolerance evaluation, which includes administering the STI (Appendix K) and possibly LDL testing (Appendix M), it then is decided if the patient should be evaluated for ear-level instruments. This decision depends largely on the extent of the problem, which should be clear after the evaluation.

Although ear-level instruments might provide the optimal treatment for a sound tolerance problem, they may not be necessary. Often, sound enrichment using a variety of sound sources can provide an adequate acoustic-desensitization protocol. The clinician should weigh the pros and cons of ear-level instruments for each patient and decide, along with the patient, if these devices might be the best choice for treatment. If so, then in-clinic trial use of ear-level instruments should be performed. The in-clinic trial can be conducted either before or after the counseling, whichever is most appropriate for the patient.

When Are Ear-Level Instruments Indicated?

The decision to use ear-level instruments with a patient who has hyperacusis is based primarily on two factors: (a) the patient's sound tolerance condition must be reasonably severe to justify the use of these instruments; and (b) the patient must be motivated to use the instruments. If either of these factors does not apply, then the patient should be counseled appropriately to use sound desensitization procedures without the use of ear-level instruments.

Conducting the In-Clinic Trial

The purpose of the in-clinic trial is to provide patients with the experience of wearing and listening to sound-generating devices—to help them decide if using ear-level instruments is desirable. The sound should be described as a "soothing shower sound" and not in negative terms such as noise or static. It is possible that some patients will not be comfortable listening to the sound, but that even just wearing the instruments might be appropriate for the first phase of treatment (i.e., some patients need to just wear the instruments turned off for a period of time before they can start listening to the sound emitted from the instruments). Conducting the trial simply is a matter of fitting each stock device to patients and allowing them to direct the process of adjusting the sound levels. This process might take more or less time depending on individual patient characteristics.

Definitions: Hyperacusis, Misophonia, Phonophobia, Loudness Recruitment

Definitions for these terms were provided in Chapter 1. They are reviewed briefly here. Hyperacusis is a physical condition of discomfort or pain caused by sound (J. A. Henry, Zaugg, et al., 2005a). The effect is restricted primarily to the auditory pathways.

Misophonia means literally "dislike of sound," implying that emotions somehow are involved in the reaction to sound (M. M. Jastreboff & P. J. Jastreboff, 2002). Misophonic reactions would be learned responses, thus the same sound might be bothersome in some situations and not in others. Phonophobia is a subcategory of misophonia, and specifically is a fear response caused by sound (P. J. Jastreboff & M. M. Jastreboff, 2000).

Any or all of these conditions might apply to a patient who complains of loudness tolerance problems. None of these conditions should be confused with loudness recruitment, which is abnormally rapid growth in the perception of loudness (Vernon, 1976). Recruitment usually is a symptom of cochlear or sensorineural hearing loss.

For purposes of PTM, any condition of reduced sound tolerance (hyperacusis, misophonia, phonophobia) is referred to as hyperacusis. The STEM program does not make a distinction between these different conditions with respect to the counseling and sound desensitization procedures. The treatment procedures are designed to address both physical and emotional aspects of reduced sound tolerance.

Conclusion

We have conducted screenings and evaluations of thousands of patients with tinnitus in multiple clinics as part of our clinical studies. It has been our experience that many of these patients report a sound tolerance problem, but that a very small number actually experience a severe problem warranting special evaluation and treatment procedures. If patients do have a severe hyperacusis problem (or if they just want treatment for reduced sound tolerance), then the STEM protocol should address their needs. The STEM protocol is implemented before the flow of PTM services continues, that is, these patients should be treated separately and then worked back into PTM as warranted by tinnitus-specific complaints.

With the STEM protocol, all patients with a severe sound tolerance problem are assumed to have some combination of hyperacusis and misophonia. Very few patients have "pure" hyperacusis or "pure" misophonia (see Chapter 1), thus a combined approach usually is appropriate. For these patients, special consideration should be given to collaborating with mental health clinicians to address potential psychological components of the problem. Behavioral interventions have been shown to be highly effective in decreasing patients' responses to intense fear. Such interventions have been well described in the CBT literature (Hofmann & Smits, 2008). Thus, psychological interventions such as CBT may be used to help patients systematically modify their fear responses, habituate to everyday sounds, and achieve a greater sense of well-being and control.

7

Level 3 Group Education

Chronic tinnitus usually is a permanent condition. In most cases tinnitus cannot be quieted, but patients can learn to manage their reactions to it. These reactions may need to be managed for a lifetime. Clinical intervention with PTM focuses on educating patients to become self-sufficient in managing their reactions to tinnitus.

This chapter provides a description of PTM Level 3 Group Education. Level 3 is the first level within the clinical hierarchy of PTM for which intervention specific to tinnitus is the primary purpose of patient visits to the clinic. During Level 2, the main focus is to evaluate and manage hearing problems, with a very brief assessment of tinnitus impact. (Fitting hearing aids at Level 2 to assist in the management of a hearing problem sometimes also results in a reduction in the impact of tinnitus, but this is not the primary purpose of fitting hearing aids at Level 2.) Intervention provided specifically for tinnitus during Level 2 is ancillary, such as answering questions and providing patients with educational materials.

Level 3 Group Education consists of a series of patient-education classes that are termed "workshops" because of their emphasis on interaction and participation. The standard protocol consists of five weekly workshops—two presented by an audiologist and three by a psychologist (or other qualified mental health provider). With respect to ordering the weekly workshops, it is recommended that the first and third workshops be those led by the audiologist, and the second, fourth, and fifth be those led by the psychologist.

The audiologist instructs patients in how sound can be used in different ways to manage reactions to tinnitus, and directs them through the process of developing individualized action plans using the Sound Plan Worksheet (Appendix N). The three workshops conducted by a psychologist provide instruction for patients to learn how to use specific coping skills to manage their reactions to tinnitus.

It should be noted that group education is not an appropriate venue for some patients, who may be unwilling to attend a group session or who may just require one-on-one intervention. Furthermore, if a patient has a cognitive impairment or other medical or mental health condition that would disrupt learning in a group education format, then the information from the groups can be discussed with the patient and his or her significant other on an individual basis.

Self-Help Workbook

In Chapters 3 and 5 we described the patient self-help workbook *How to Manage Your Tinnitus: A Step-by-Step Workbook* (J. A. Henry et al., 2010a). The workbook is fairly comprehensive in that it provides a great deal of information to guide patients in learning how to self-manage their reactions to tinnitus. We have recommended that patients who participate in Level 3 Group Education receive a copy of the workbook when they attend their first workshop. In Chapter 5, we described reasons for waiting until Level 3 to provide the workbook. In general, it will be more effective for patients when used in conjunction with their participation in the workshops.

Collaborative Self-Management

As explained in Chapter 3, when referring to intervention for chronic tinnitus, we do not use the word "treatment," which can imply that a provider performs some procedure (or administers a drug) that is intended to quiet the tinnitus of a patient who passively receives the procedure. We instead adhere to the notion that intervention should primarily involve educating the patient about *managing reactions* to tinnitus. Different strategies often are needed to manage reactions to tinnitus that occur in different situations. Patients need to learn these strategies so they can manage any life experience disrupted by the symptom. This learning should take place with a compassionate and knowledgeable clinician who provides the education.

The PTM approach to self-management is modeled closely after clinical methodologies recently developed for chronic pain management (Blyth, March, Nicholas, & Cousins, 2005). In the past, urgent pain relief depended on treatments such as opioid drugs or invasive surgeries. It now is recognized that effective management of chronic pain depends much more on patients' own efforts and expectations than on their passively receiving a treatment. In essence, biomedical solutions are being supplanted by educational approaches that focus on supporting long-term rehabilitation.

As patients become more actively involved in decisions affecting their clinical care, they naturally experience a greater sense of commitment to participate in the management process. This results in "a shift of responsibility from the health-care professional to the individual for the day-to-day management of their condition" (S. Newman, Mulligan, & Steed, 2001) (p. 1). Accomplishing this "shift of responsibility" requires working with patients to help them: (a) understand their condition; (b) participate in decisions regarding their management plan; (c) develop and follow the plan; and (d) monitor success of their self-management efforts and revise the plan as needed. The clinician and patient should maintain a therapeutic relationship, with contacts occurring either on an "as needed" or periodic basis (i.e., regular follow-ups). This overall approach appropriately is termed "collaborative self-management."

Educating Patients to Use Therapeutic Sound

The use of therapeutic sound for tinnitus management is well supported clinically and by clinical research (J. A. Henry et al., 2008c). Evidence for sound-based tinnitus management has been reported for tinnitus masking (Folmer & Carroll, 2006; Hazell et al., 1985; Schleuning et al., 1980; Stephens & Corcoran, 1985), tinnitus retraining therapy (Bartnik et al., 2001; Berry et al., 2002; Herraiz et al., 2005; Herraiz et al., 2007), and neuromonics tinnitus treatment (P. B. Davis et al., 2007). In addition, hearing aids are well known to provide benefit for patients with tinnitus (Del Bo & Ambrosetti, 2007; Folmer & Carroll, 2006; Saltzman & Ersner, 1947; Surr et al., 1999; Surr et al., 1985; Trotter & Donaldson, 2008).

We completed two prospective clinical trials that involved fitting hearing aids, ear-level noise generators, or combination instruments to most of the subjects (see "First Study" and "Third Study" in Chapter 2). All cohorts, regardless of the specific intervention involved, showed significant improvement (to varying degrees). Folmer and Carroll (2006) evaluated long-term outcomes in OHSU Tinnitus Clinic patients. Three groups of 50 patients each were evaluated who: (a) used ear-level noise generators; (b) used hearing aids; and (c) did not use ear-level devices. Although significant improvement was observed for all patients, those who used ear-level devices experienced significantly better outcomes than those who did not use devices.

An abundance of studies and clinical techniques support the use of therapeutic sound to manage tinnitus. It is important to note, however, that no one method has been shown to be superior over the others. With PTM, patients are not limited to a single method or a particular device. Rather, the approach is to provide patients with the knowledge and skills to use sound and sound devices in adaptive ways to manage any life situation disrupted by tinnitus. This is accomplished by teaching patients the different ways that sound can be used to manage reactions to tinnitus, and helping them develop and implement custom sound-based management plans that address their unique needs.

Workshops Conducted by an Audiologist

As mentioned above, Level 3 Group Education ideally consists of two workshops facilitated by an audiologist and three by a mental health provider. A PowerPoint presentation (*Managing Your Tinnitus: What to Do and How to Do It*) is given during each workshop (the two PowerPoint presentations made by audiologists are provided on the CD that is included with this handbook). The leader makes the presentations, facilitates discussion, and addresses any questions or concerns. The focus of the two Level 3 classes facilitated by an audiologist is to assist patients in learning how to self-manage their reactions to tinnitus using therapeutic sound in adaptive ways.

First Workshop (With Audiologist)

The goal for session one is for all group participants to use the Sound Plan Worksheet (see Appendix N) to develop an individualized "sound plan" for managing their most bothersome tinnitus situation. It is essential that participants learn how to use the worksheet to organize their efforts for using therapeutic sound.

The focus of education with PTM is to provide patients with practical, how-to information. The group sessions thus are task-oriented so the time must be spent teaching the participants what to *do* to manage their reactions to tinnitus. Covering all of the structured material during each session requires up to an hour and a half. Keeping these groups on-task can be challenging. There is a natural tendency for patients to want to share their experiences and thoughts about tinnitus, and they have limited opportunity to do that during the sessions. Also, any discussion about tinnitus inevitably leads to many questions. For these reasons, participants are asked to refrain from asking questions and discussing topics unrelated to the workshop until the end of the session. Discussion and questions relevant to the topics being presented are encouraged.

Review the Tinnitus and Hearing Survey

Prior to enrollment in group education, each participant should have filled out the Tinnitus and Hearing Survey (THS; Appendix D). As described in Chapter 5, the THS is designed to assist patients and clinicians in understanding how much of a patient's problem is due to tinnitus and how much is due to hearing problems. It is critical for participants to have used the THS to determine candidacy for enrollment in Level 3 Group Education. In Chapter 5, a list of requirements was provided that should be used to ensure that a patient's participation in Level 3 is appropriate.

If group participants do not bring their completed THS to the session, then they should complete one at the start of the session. The THS is then reviewed during the session—the concepts are discussed and participants are asked to share their responses on the THS. This is done to ensure that all participants understand that the purpose of the classes is to address tinnitus-specific problems and that problems related to hearing are not addressed during the workshops.

Sound Plan Worksheet

Use of the Sound Plan Worksheet (see Appendix N) facilitates the process of identifying sounds and sound-generating devices that are expected to be effective in managing specific tinnitus-problem situations. The worksheet is used throughout the first session with the objective for each participant to develop a "sound plan" that will be used until the second session to manage the participant's "most bothersome" tinnitus situation. After participants have gained experience and confidence with the process and the concepts of developing sound plans, then additional bothersome tinnitus situations can be addressed and more complicated and sophisticated technology can be incorporated. Participants are encouraged to use the worksheet on a regular basis to refine and improve their sound plans.

Creating a sound plan to address one problem situation involves four small tasks (No. 1 to 4 on the Sound Plan Worksheet) that likely can be accomplished successfully by patients: (1) identify a situation when tinnitus is problematic; (2) determine which strategy (or strategies) for using sound will be implemented in that situation; (3) determine a specific sound that will be used with each strategy; and (4) determine a specific device for presenting each sound. The plan is used for at least one week and then evaluated for its effectiveness (No. 5 on the worksheet).

Group participants are instructed to identify, using the Tinnitus Problem Checklist (see Appendix H), the life situation in which their tinnitus is the "most bothersome." To increase the likelihood that the initial sound plan will be implemented successfully, they then create a sound plan to manage just that one situation using sounds and sound devices that are readily accessible. In this way, participants are empowered in creating a sound plan that can be implemented with minimal effort and usually at no cost to address their most bothersome tinnitus situation.

Three Types of Sound

To complete the Sound Plan Worksheet, participants must learn about the three types of sound (soothing, interesting, and background) that can be used to manage reactions to tinnitus. The three types of sound have been described in detail elsewhere (J. A. Henry et al., 2008c), and are reviewed briefly below.

Soothing Sound. Soothing sound is any sound that provides an immediate sense of relief from stress or tension that is caused by tinnitus. The use of soothing sound has its roots in the method of tinnitus masking, which originally was described by Vernon (1976). The method of tinnitus masking continues to be used, and relies on the use of ear-level "maskers" that generate broadband noise (Schechter & J. A. Henry, 2002). The use of sound with tinnitus masking is intended to provide an immediate sense of relief—not to "mask" tinnitus, as the name would seem to imply.

Soothing sound for tinnitus management is not restricted to the use of ear-level maskers and broadband noise. Any sound that produces a sense of relief (or that the patient considers soothing) can be used as soothing sound. When using soothing sound, it is important that patients focus on obtaining a sense of relief from stress and tension rather than focusing on how much their tinnitus is masked. We therefore decided to abandon use of the term "masking" altogether. Whether or not the tinnitus is masked is completely irrelevant to the use of soothing sound.

Interesting Sound. Interesting sound is used to actively divert attention away from the tinnitus. The use of interesting sound for tinnitus management has not been a part of any formal method of therapy for tinnitus. However, distraction is a concept that is used for pain management, and the use of interesting sound follows the basic pain model (M. H. Johnson, 2005). In essence, using interesting sound to manage reactions to tinnitus is intended to shift the patient's attention away from the tinnitus and onto some other sound. Patients thus learn to "actively listen" to sounds that they find interesting or entertaining, which accomplishes the distraction objective.

Background Sound. Some patients do not experience a satisfactory sense of relief from sound and so may be tempted to abandon its use altogether. It is important that patients understand that even if sound does not provide immediate relief (or if it is not interesting), it still can be very effective in managing reactions to tinnitus by reducing the contrast between tinnitus and the acoustic environment, thereby making it easier for the brain to let the tinnitus go unnoticed.

The "candle in a dark room" analogy is used to demonstrate the concept behind background sound (as shown on the video that is provided with this handbook). A burning candle in a dark room naturally attracts attention because of the high contrast between the flame and the dark surroundings. If the room is then lighted, the contrast is reduced causing the flame to attract less attention—even though it has not changed. This analogy helps patients to understand the purpose of using background sound.

The use of background sound for tinnitus management is derived from the method of tinnitus retraining therapy (TRT) (P. J. Jastreboff & Hazell, 2004), which started as a clinical technique in the late 1980s. The method continues to be used and relies on the use of sound to promote "habituation" (decrease in responsiveness) to tinnitus reactions and perception. Patients with more severe tinnitus are advised to use ear-level sound generators (or combination instruments). These patients are instructed to adjust the level of the broadband noise to below the "mixing point," that is, below the level at which their tinnitus sound starts to change (J. A. Henry, Trune, et al., 2007a). Many of our patients and research participants had difficulty adjusting the sound to the mixing point, and often seemed generally confused and sometimes anxious about the mixing-point concept. The use of background sound is intended to accomplish essentially the same purpose as for TRT. However, we do not refer to the mixing point, habituation, or other terminology that is specific to TRT. In this way, patients learn what to do but are not expected to adhere to a protocol that can seem complicated and daunting to accomplish. Patients certainly are encouraged to learn more about the TRT concepts if they are interested.

Demonstrating the Three Types of Sound

Specific activities were developed to give group participants the opportunity to experience each of the three types of sound. Visual scales are provided to enhance understanding of the activities (J. A. Henry et al., 2008c). The visual scales are demonstrated to participants during the first session so that they can appreciate their utility. Participants learn that they can use the tools on their own to evaluate the effectiveness of different sounds for ongoing tinnitus management.

The Relief Scale (Appendix O) was developed as a tool for PTM patients to use to (a) learn how soothing sound is used to manage reactions to tinnitus, and (b) identify sounds and evaluate their ability to induce relief. Patients listen to the demonstration sound and then answer the question, "How much relief do I feel?" The six-point response scale ranges from "no relief" (no reduction in stress or tension caused by tinnitus) to "complete relief" (elimination of stress or tension caused by tinnitus). Participants are asked to share their ratings with the group.

The Attention Scale (Appendix P) was developed for use during an activity in which patients learn how interesting sound can divert attention away from tinnitus. The scale is used as a tool to help patients identify the kinds of sounds that most effectively shift their thoughts away from the tinnitus. Patients are instructed to select any sound or sound passage that they would expect to keep their attention. After listening to the sound for at least one minute, they estimate the percentage of attention focused on the "interesting" sound versus the tinnitus. A sound passage is played during the workshop to demonstrate interesting sound, and participants are asked to share their ratings on the Attention Scale with the group.

The notion of reducing auditory contrast between tinnitus and sound in the environment can be demonstrated to participants using a visual analog. Tinnitus in a quiet environment results in high contrast. The addition of sound reduces the contrast. Patients can hear this effect by first noticing how their tinnitus sounds in quiet, and then adding sound. The Tinnitus Contrast Activity (Appendix Q) serves as a visual analog to facilitate demonstrating this effect. Patients use the Tinnitus Contrast Activity while listening to different sounds. Although each sound reduces contrast by a different amount, patients are taught that any amount of contrast reduction can be beneficial—provided the sound is experienced at a comfortable level. One or more background sounds are demonstrated to the group, and participants are asked to relate the concept depicted by the analog to the effect that is achieved with the sound.

Sound Grid

For each of the three *types* of sound (soothing, background, interesting), environmental sound, music, and speech can be used. This results in nine possible combinations, as shown by the sound grid (Figure 7–1). *Environmental sound* includes any nature sound (sounds of animals, weather, moving water, etc.) or synthetic (manmade) sound (e.g., electric fans and appliances, broadband masking noise, synthesized sounds). *Music* of all styles can be used, including music with and without lyrics. *Speech* of all varieties is appropriate to utilize, including lectures, sermons, talk radio, guided imagery, crowd noise, one-on-one conversation, and so forth.

Case Example

A case example demonstrates how patients use the Sound Plan Worksheet (please refer to Appendix N). Mr. Roberts' most bothersome situation was "being annoyed by his tinnitus while working in his quiet office" (No. 1). As a general strategy (No. 2), he thought that using background sound might in general be helpful. The specific sound he would try would be constant fan noise (No. 3) from a small fan in his office (No. 4). He tried this plan for one week and determined that the plan was "a little" helpful (No. 5). He then revised his plan by adding soothing sound (No. 2). He liked sounds of nature and decided to listen to beach sounds (No. 3) using a CD and CD player that he already owned (No. 4). After trying a combination of fan noise and sounds of nature for one week, he indicated that the plan helped him "a lot" (No. 5). Mr. Roberts' initial sound plan demonstrated limited success. Based on that experience, he revised his plan and the new plan worked well for him. He experienced success using the worksheet to address one particular problem situation, and he now uses the worksheet as needed to develop plans to address other problem situations.

	Environmental	Music	Speech
Soothing	✓	✓	✓
Background	✓	✓	✓
Interesting	✓	✓	✓

Figure 7–1. Sound grid. This grid shows that there are three *types* of sound (soothing, background, interesting) that can be used to manage reactions to tinnitus. Each type of sound can involve the use of environmental sound, music, and/or speech to manage specific tinnitus-problem situations. A total of nine combinations of sound are possible as indicated by the nine checkmarks.

Second Workshop (With Audiologist)

At the end of the first workshop, group participants are asked to return for a follow-up workshop two weeks later. Between workshops, their "homework" is to carry out and evaluate the effectiveness of their initial sound plan. Participants should bring their worksheet developed at the first session to the second session. They are told that they can modify the plan during the second session to improve its effectiveness.

The objectives of the second workshop are for participants to: (a) share their experiences using their initial sound plan; (b) engage in collaborative problem solving (to address any problems implementing their sound plans); and (c) improve their sound plan or develop a new sound plan. In addition, new information is covered during the second workshop, including descriptions of: (a) different types of sound-producing devices; (b) ideas for using sound to improve sleep; (c) sound-based methods of tinnitus management and how they relate to the sound grid (see Figure 7–1); and (d) lifestyle factors that can affect tinnitus and hearing. Participants should attend both workshops to maximize their benefit. Participants who attend only the first workshop should receive follow-up by telephone.

Workshops Conducted by a Psychologist

Mental health intervention can be an important component of an overall approach to managing tinnitus for all patients. Patients who are bothered by tinnitus can, in general, benefit from receiving mental health intervention to alter maladaptive reactions to tinnitus and to aid in coping with tinnitus. Mental health intervention is particularly important for patients with tinnitus who also experience post-traumatic stress disorder (PTSD), depression, anxiety, or other mental health problems.

A major question in the development of CBT for Level 3 was the number of sessions that should be conducted. Six to ten sessions of CBT are typical in many clinical settings. The actual number of CBT sessions is flexible, however, and depends on the purpose of the therapy. Beck (1995) explained that "Most straight-forward patients with depression and anxiety disorders are treated for 4 to 14 sessions" (p. 7). One controlled study has shown that a condensed version of CBT for tinnitus can be conducted in two sessions with no differences in disability reduction relative to a group that attended 11 sessions (Kroner-Herwig, Frenzel, Fritsche, Schilkowsky, & Esser, 2003). Consistent with a "progressive" approach to tinnitus management, patients should receive less intervention at lower levels and more intervention at higher levels. Therefore only certain components of CBT are taught at Level 3 so as to minimize the number of sessions that patients are expected to attend at this level of care.

We determined that three CBT sessions at Level 3 would be necessary to cover the most important components of CBT (described below). Patients then have the option of attending additional sessions if further CBT counseling is needed. These additional sessions normally are offered to patients following, and depending on the results of the Level 4 Interdisciplinary Evaluation. In addition, the Level 3 protocol is flexible such that if multiple participants in the CBT workshops require additional intervention, then additional workshops can be added—which again is consistent with the progressive approach.

Typically, in CBT when basic information about the problem is provided, this is called psychoeducation and usually is presented during the first session of CBT. The last session of CBT typically includes information about preventing the problem from recurring or getting worse. For example, when CBT is used to treat depression, during the last session patients normally are taught how to identify early signs of depression relapse (such as overeating) or how to prevent depression (such as exercising regularly). Psychoeducation and planning for flare-ups and exposure to loud noise during PTM is presented in the self-help workbook provided to each patient, and thus, this information is not repeated during the Level 3 CBT workshops with the mental health provider. Consequently, more than three sessions of CBT would create some redundancies using the PTM structure. However, all information (basics of CBT, psychoeducation, protecting hearing, and flare-up planning) and the CBT skills addressing stress reduction, attention diversion, and cognitive restructuring are reviewed if the patient progresses to Level 5 Individualized Support.

Patient learning in all of the Level 3 workshops is facilitated by use of the PTM self-help workbook (J. A. Henry, Zaugg, Myers, & Kendall, 2010a). Each of the CBT components taught during Level 3 is described in the workbook. After each session, patients practice their new skills by using worksheets and activities in the workbook. These worksheets and activities are intended to facilitate learning the new skills and recording progress. When patients return for the next workshop, they are asked to report their progress to the group. Group education based on CBT, as opposed to individual CBT sessions, is efficient and allows patients to apply skills to a variety of situations and to develop a social network from which to draw support.

Changing Thoughts and Feelings Worksheet

During the CBT workshops the Changing Thoughts and Feelings Worksheet is used, which is modeled after and used simultaneously with the Sound Plan Worksheet (see Appendix N). The Changing Thoughts and Feelings Worksheet helps patients track their use of the three coping skills offered during the CBT portion of Level 3. The worksheets are used throughout the sessions with the objective for participants to develop personalized plans for managing their reactions to tinnitus in specific problem-situations.

CBT group participants are instructed to identify, using the Tinnitus Problem Checklist (see Appendix H), the life situation in which their tinnitus is the "most bothersome." This is the same task that is required when they use the Sound Plan Worksheet during the workshops conducted by an audiologist. It is helpful if patients identify the same tinnitus problem on their two different worksheets to learn how very different strategies can be used to address a single problem situation. The audiologists and mental health providers who teach these workshops should point this out and ask participants to focus first on their most bothersome tinnitus problem. In the process, patients learn that managing reactions to tinnitus involves using a combination of strategies that each are developed and refined through trial and error. Learning to manage tinnitus is a process that should be conducted systematically—by learning the strategies, developing action plans, implementing the plans, and revising the plans to improve outcomes.

After the group participants have gained experience and confidence with the process and the use of CBT concepts to manage their reactions to tinnitus, they can use any of the skills as "tools" to help them cope with their tinnitus. They are encouraged to use the Thoughts and Feelings Worksheet on a regular basis to refine and improve their use of these coping skills.

Essential CBT Components

The Level 3 workshops led by a mental health provider focus on teaching three CBT techniques: stress reduction ("relaxation"), attention diversion ("planning pleasant activities"), and cognitive restructuring ("changing thoughts"). During the first CBT session, the basic premise that how one thinks and acts influences one's feelings is described. Emphasis is placed on clarifying goals and tracking efforts. Later, patients learn techniques to assist them in learning ways to modify thoughts and increase or decrease behaviors that influence how they feel about their tinnitus. Each of these coping skills can be helpful to patients who want to learn ways to manage their reactions to tinnitus. These skills also are applicable to many other chronic conditions such as anxiety, depression, and pain.

CBT Session I

Stress Reduction

Many patients report that their tinnitus is exacerbated by stress. By reducing stress or managing reactions to stress, patients are able to reset the body's natural stress arousal system to a more relaxed and calm state. Practicing relaxation techniques can modify one's response to stress and can serve to distract attention from the tinnitus to other things. The goal of providing this skill is to empower patients with a simple and easy way to relax when stressed.

Relaxation techniques taught during the first session of Level 3 with the psychologist include controlled breathing and imagery. A video demonstration of these techniques ("Deep Breathing" and "Imagery") is included on the DVD that is provided with the self-help workbook. The "Deep Breathing" exercise is a controlled breathing exercise that helps patients focus on taking slow and rhythmic breaths. Controlled breathing encourages attention to the mechanisms of the lungs and sounds of breathing, which releases tension and diverts attention from tinnitus. The "Imagery" exercise teaches patients to imagine being somewhere calming and safe. Imagery is useful as a relaxation technique when a pleasant or neutral image is envisioned during distress (J. L. Henry & Wilson, 2001). These techniques also require practice, thus, patients are asked to complete "homework" between sessions.

Instructions for both of these relaxation exercises are specific for patients with tinnitus. For example, patients are instructed not to practice the relaxation exercises in silence. Patients are encouraged to use soothing sound such as calming music during the exercises. Furthermore, since many patients with tinnitus also have hearing loss, instructions take into account the fact that some patients may feel more comfortable not closing their eyes during the relaxation exercises. They are instructed to focus on an object in the room or on the open-captioning of the relaxation demonstrations on the video.

Attention Diversion via Increasing Pleasant Activities

There are many ways to divert attention from one activity to another. Many patients stop doing the things they like to do (pleasant activities) and tend to focus on required activities such as work and house chores. The goal of providing this coping skill is to help patients learn ways to divert attention away from the tinnitus and onto other things by increasing pleasant activities in their lives. This skill also is taught during the first session of Level 3 with the mental health provider. The skill typically is easy for patients to understand.

Group participants are instructed to examine the impact of tinnitus on their activities, particularly on pleasant activities, and to learn ways to increase their activities. They are provided a list of types of activities (solitary, indoor, social, musical, etc.) from which to develop ideas about the types of activities they would enjoy. They then are asked to add one pleasant activity to their daily routine and rate how effective it was in diverting attention away from the tinnitus.

Increasing activities helps to distract patients from their tinnitus and helps them to gain meaningful experiences that typically result in a greater sense of relatedness and connectedness to the world. Also, patients may have become isolated over the course of learning to cope with their tinnitus. Some patients will need encouragement to become social again.

CBT Sessions 2 and 3: Cognitive Restructuring

During the second and third CBT workshops, the group participants are taught how their thoughts and behaviors influence feelings via a step-by-step guide for evaluating thoughts, modifying thoughts, and developing healthy attitudes. These cognitive restructuring activities require two sessions to adequately cover all the material.

CBT Session 2

During the first of the two sessions on cognitive restructuring, participants learn about healthy attitudes and examining their own thoughts; this sometimes is called "mindfulness" training. Mindfulness is a state of being consciously aware of one's own thoughts and behaviors. Some patients tend to use faulty logic when thinking about experiences.

During this session, participants learn the 12 most common types of negative appraisals (also called thought errors): (1) overgeneralization, (2) all-or-none thinking, (3) filtering or selective abstraction, (4) mind-reading, (5) magnification or catastrophization, (6) minimization, (7) personalization, (8) jumping to conclusions or arbitrary inference, (9) emotional reasoning, (10) "should" statements, (11) labeling, and (12) blaming (Beck, 1995). They are taught to be mindful by systematically examining their thoughts so as to provide insight into which of these 12 negative appraisals they may be using. They are asked to cite personal examples for each of the 12 negative appraisals as homework. As they do this exercise, thought patterns or "habits" typically emerge, helping them understand their own thought processes.

CBT Session 3

During the second of the two sessions on cognitive restructuring, the participants learn to systematically modify or restructure their thoughts so as to create different, more desirable emotional reactions. Constructive approaches to stress, such as thinking of a stressful event as a challenge rather than a threat, are presented. Negative attitudes and appraisals of situations often lead to negative emotions, which immediately are applied to individuals' unique problems and concerns.

During this session, step-by-step instructions are provided for changing negative appraisals to more constructive, positive appraisals. The group works through an example in their workbook of using the step-by-step process to address a negative thought about an event and come up with alternative, more constructive thoughts. The participants' life situation in which their tinnitus is most bothersome as identified on the Tinnitus Problem Checklist (see Appendix H) is used during this exercise to keep the CBT sessions aligned with the sessions with the audiologist.

Post-Workshop Follow-Up

Patients who attend the workshops should be informed that they will receive a follow-up phone call approximately one month after the last workshop. The call is made by the audiologist or the mental health provider who conducted the workshops. The purpose of the call is to determine if the patient will return for the Level 4 Interdisciplinary Evaluation. During the call, the clinician asks about progress implementing the action plans, discusses any problems encountered, and answers questions. The clinician can use any of the written questionnaires that were administered previously to assist in determining if a Level 4 appointment is warranted.

Conclusion

Any person who has tinnitus can benefit from being educated concerning what to do about the phantom sound. Many patients are interested only in a cure for their tinnitus, and they may not realize the importance of learning good management techniques. In general, clinical services for tinnitus are provided only to patients who are *bothered* by their tinnitus. The majority of individuals who experience tinnitus are not bothered by the constant sound and they mainly need to learn and adhere to good practices to avoid situations that can damage their hearing. Those who *are* bothered by their tinnitus need to learn methods to self-manage their reactions to tinnitus. With PTM, these methods include education about using therapeutic sound and effective coping techniques.

The goals of PTM are achieved through the process of *collaborative* self-management. Clinicians who provide PTM should consider themselves as a source of information and support that empowers patients to manage any situation in which tinnitus is problematic. As already discussed, collaborative self-management is very different from the traditional "treatment" model, which involves patients passively undergoing some kind of therapeutic procedure(s). The keys to collaborative self-management are the availability of appropriate educational materials and the means to provide the education to patients efficiently and effectively. The framework of PTM provides for a variety of modalities through which patients can learn the essential self-help information. Level 3 Group Education is sufficient for most patients who are bothered by tinnitus. If further services are required, then the patient should be scheduled for a Level 4 Interdisciplinary Evaluation, which is described in the next chapter.

8

Level 4 Interdisciplinary Evaluation

Most patients can satisfactorily self-manage their reactions to tinnitus after participating in Level 3 Group Education. Patients who need more support and education than is available at Level 3 can progress to the Level 4 Interdisciplinary Evaluation, which normally includes evaluations by an audiologist and a mental health provider who is trained to conduct psychological assessments.

The main purpose of the Level 4 Interdisciplinary Evaluation is to determine if individualized clinical services are needed to address tinnitus-specific problems. If these services are needed, then patients progress to Level 5 Individualized Support. Level 5 involves primarily one-on-one counseling from an audiologist (using the counseling book *Progressive Tinnitus Management: Counseling Guide*; J. A. Henry et al., 2010b) and/or a mental health provider. The audiologic counseling information essentially is the same as what is covered during the Level 3 workshops. However, the individualized format of the Level 5 counseling allows more personalized interaction and support than can be provided during Level 3. Level 5 intervention offered by a mental health provider includes further enhancement of skills for coping with tinnitus (taught during Level 3) such as additional relaxation techniques, attention control, and planning for "flare-ups."

The audiologic assessment that is conducted as part of the Level 4 Interdisciplinary Evaluation involves conducting a structured interview and can include, as optional procedures, a tinnitus psychoacoustic assessment and/or evaluation for use of sound therapy devices. Administration of the Tinnitus and Hearing Survey (see Appendix D) in conjunction with the Tinnitus Interview (Appendix R) is the primary means of determining if one-on-one individualized support is appropriate. If so, then the audiologist and patient begin to formulate a management plan. Special procedures are used to evaluate and select ear-level devices for tinnitus management, including hearing aids, noise/sound generators, and combination instruments.

Mental Health Assessment

Systematic progression through the different levels of PTM effectively ensures that patients reaching the Level 4 Interdisciplinary Evaluation have a severe tinnitus problem that warrants an in-depth evaluation to determine if individualized support is appropriate. Due to the severity of their distress from tinnitus, these patients also are more likely to have comorbid mental health conditions or sleep disorders that would require an interdisciplinary approach to intervention. Screening for mental health conditions and sleep disorders therefore is conducted routinely by a mental health provider as part of the Level 4 evaluation (unless the patient was recently evaluated/diagnosed by a mental health professional and currently is receiving care accordingly).

If a mental health provider is included in the facility's "tinnitus team," then that individual should conduct the mental health assessment. Full assessment of mental health symptoms should be conducted by someone qualified to do such an evaluation such as a psychologist or psychiatrist. If a mental health provider is not part of the team, then the patient should be referred to primary care for a mental health assessment (or referred as dictated by the facility's referral procedures). Finally, as discussed next, a nonmental health provider can conduct mental health screening in certain situations. However, those situations should be rare, as timely and collaborative mental health services are available within most health care organizations.

Mental Health Screening by Nonmental Health Clinicians

It is best for mental health screening to be performed by a psychologist or other mental health care provider who is familiar with the effects of hearing loss and tinnitus. If such a provider is unavailable, then basic screening for these symptoms can be conducted by any clinician who has been properly trained to use screening tools and who has resources for responding to their outcomes. In instances where audiologists (or other nonmental health care providers) are performing screening for referral to mental health, collaborations with mental health are essential to allow for immediate referrals and follow-up as warranted. Hospitals and outpatient clinics vary in the types and availability of mental health clinicians. When appropriate mental health care providers are unavailable, primary care providers often can be helpful as many have training and experience with screening for sleep and mental health problems.

Nonmental health clinicians must be cautious in dealing with any issues related to anxiety, depression, stress disorders, suicidality or suicidal thoughts, risky behavior, and so forth, because this is not their area of expertise. These clinicians must use the mental health screening tools only to aid in making appropriate referrals, and cannot provide diagnostic interpretation of test scores. Some patients may feel uncomfortable with these types of questions, or that the questioning is inappropriate and intrusive. Therefore, it is important to ask for permission to explore these issues, for example, "If you don't mind, I would like to ask you some questions about your mood and things that can affect your mood. Sometimes ringing in the ears is made worse when other conditions are present at the same time."

Before formally screening for mental health conditions, it is helpful to start with the patient's medical records and scan for comorbid conditions that previously have been identified. After reviewing the chart, there are several options for identifying a need for referral to a different discipline. Simple mental health screeners can be useful in determining if a referral to a mental health clinician is warranted. Screening instruments are available to screen for anxiety, depression, and PTSD—the mental health conditions that have been observed to co-occur most commonly in patients who complain of bothersome tinnitus. Each medical facility has its preferred mental health screening tools and protocols. It is best to contact a mental health clinician or primary care physician at your site in advance to learn which screening tools are recommended for use by audiologists. Some sites prefer to funnel all mental health screenings into one service where an intake appointment is made to determine the needs of all referred patients. In some settings, health services are centralized to primary care providers (PCPs). Thus, it might be necessary to refer a patient to a PCP when there is any suspicion of a mental health or sleep disorder. The PCP then assesses the appropriateness of referral to a mental health or sleep clinic. At many sites audiologists must take the lead in educating other professionals about PTM and the interdisciplinary nature of this methodology.

A basic mental health screening battery can be completed in about 10 to 15 minutes. The results can assist in determining the potential need to involve other disciplines in the patient's clinical management. Further assessment of these conditions is performed by a mental health provider as indicated by results of the screening tests.

Anxiety and Depression

Screening for anxiety and depression can be performed using the Hospital Anxiety and Depression Scale (HADS—Appendix S) (Zigmond & Snaith, 1983). This self-screening questionnaire consists of 14 questions—seven for anxiety and seven for depression. Patients should be instructed to complete this self-screening questionnaire by responding *spontaneously* to each item. The HADS has been used extensively in primary care settings (Wilkinson & Barczak, 1988).

Post-Traumatic Stress Disorder

The Primary Care PTSD screening tool (PC-PTSD) (Prins et al., 2004) is available to detect possible PTSD, and to initiate appropriate referral (Appendix T). The PC-PTSD was designed for use in primary care and other medical settings and currently is used widely to screen for PTSD in military veterans. The four-item instrument enables rapid screening with high sensitivity but low specificity. The PC-PTSD is effective for capturing patients who require further evaluation for possible PTSD (although patients can have active symptoms and screen negative).

Other Mental Health Conditions

The disorder-specific screening tools that are recommended (HADS and PC-PTSD) address mental health disorders that have been observed commonly to co-occur with tinnitus. Use of these tools, however, does not adequately address the range of other mental health problems that can exist in these patients (see Chapter 5). Another approach to screening for mental health problems is to use a symptom checklist, which often is included as part of general intake questionnaires in medical clinics. Use of a symptom checklist might reduce a patient's perceived stigma of mental health problems. Systematic screening using screening tools or checklists can be helpful, but is not necessary to justify referring a patient to a provider of a different discipline. The reason for referral often is simply that the clinician perceives that there are problems outside his or her field of expertise.

Sleep Disorders

As discussed in Chapter 5, sleep disorders are the most common problem reported by patients seeking clinical services for tinnitus, especially those with the most severe tinnitus problem. A brief questionnaire is available to screen patients for sleep disorders: the Epworth Sleepiness Scale (ESS—Appendix U) (Johns, 1991). The ESS is the most widely used standardized tool for assessing "sleepiness." Completing the ESS provides an index score that can be compared to normative data. A score of 10 or more on the ESS suggests that the patient is not getting adequate sleep (for any reason), and may need to be referred to a physician for an evaluation.

In addition to insomnia, there are many other categories of sleep disorders. These include difficulty initiating and maintaining sleep, and sleep-phase disorders. These disorders usually are behaviorally based, responsive to behavioral interventions, and do not necessarily require specialty care (although sleep-phase disorders are best evaluated by a sleep clinic).

More serious categories of sleep disorder include sleep apneas and sleep-disordered breathing, REM behavior disorders, and narcolepsy. These can be serious medical conditions (especially sleep-disordered breathing, which can increase the risk of stroke) that warrant medical treatment with medications or other devices. Screening for sleep apneas/sleep-disordered breathing usually includes questions about snoring, morning headaches, waking with gasping or choking, and asking if a bed partner notices any of these things. People with sleep apnea often spend sufficient time sleeping but still do not feel rested in the morning. Sleep apneas and sleep-disordered breathing, REM behavior disorders, and narcolepsy generally are very pronounced and are conditions that usually are not related to tinnitus. Tinnitus-related insomnia generally does not necessitate referral to a sleep clinic unless the patient also reports symptoms of sleep-disordered breathing (snoring, morning headaches, etc.).

If a sleep disorder is due primarily to the patient reacting to tinnitus when attempting to sleep, then implementing the strategies offered by PTM may be sufficient to restore normal sleep patterns (see Chapter 5—Managing Sleep Disorder). Therapeutic sound can be highly effective in the sleep environment. Patients should learn the different combinations of using sound to optimize the potential for therapeutic sound to be helpful. These patients also may benefit from learning basic information about sleep hygiene such as limiting daytime napping, keeping a regular sleep schedule, and other behaviors that encourage sleep. In the PTM self-help workbook (J. A. Henry et al., 2010a) Appendix I provides three pages of "tips for getting better sleep."

Re-Administer Written Questionnaires at Level 4

Every patient who attends the Level 4 Interdisciplinary Evaluation should have completed all testing that normally is done at the Level 2 Audiologic Evaluation. At the Level 2 appointment, patients completed the Tinnitus and Hearing Survey (see Appendix D), Tinnitus Handicap Inventory (see Appendix F), and Hearing Handicap Inventory (see Appendix G). Patients should complete each of these written questionnaires again at the Level 4 appointment with the audiologist. Readministering these questionnaires enables a comparison of responses between the Level 2 and Level 4 appointments, which can reveal any longitudinal changes in a patient's self-perception of hearing and/or tinnitus handicap. The information obtained from the written questionnaires comprises an important component of the Level 4 evaluation. The structured interview would be incomplete without this information.

Administer the Tinnitus Interview

Although the use of written tinnitus questionnaires is advocated for all tinnitus patients, these questionnaires are insufficient for patients who reach Level 4. A supplemental tinnitus-specific interview (Tinnitus Interview—see Appendix R), which facilitates face-to-face structured dialogue with the patient, is necessary to capture the information needed to make decisions for clinical services at this level and helps to build rapport between patient and clinician. The patient's responses to the Tinnitus and Hearing Survey (THS) in conjunction with the Tinnitus Interview are the most important components of the audiologic portion of the Level 4 Interdisciplinary Evaluation. The interview offers a uniform format for asking questions and for recording responses. It should be completed in about 45 minutes, although its time of administration can vary considerably depending mostly on the extent of the patient's problems.

The Tinnitus Interview is designed to supplement the THS during Level 4—*it is not a stand-alone interview*. Results of the THS should first be reviewed with the patient, after which the interview can be administered if appropriate. Reviewing the THS results provides both the patient and clinician with a good understanding of the patient's current perception of problems with tinnitus, hearing, and loudness tolerance. This discussion gives the clinician opportunity to explain to the patient the types of intervention available for each of these auditory problems.

If it is confirmed that the patient has a tinnitus-specific problem and is interested in tinnitus-specific intervention, then the next step is to conduct the Tinnitus Interview. It should be noted that the Tinnitus Interview does not cover information that most likely was discussed during the case history performed during the Level 2 Audiologic Evaluation. The case history normally would obtain a description of the tinnitus (loudness, pitch, timbre, perceived location, symmetry/asymmetry, constancy versus intermittency, and so on) and the circumstances of its onset. It may be helpful to review the case history before administering the Tinnitus Interview. However, it is important not to focus on what the tinnitus sounds like since the purpose of intervention is to assist the patient in learning how to manage reactions to tinnitus—not to attempt to change the sound of the tinnitus.

Question 1: Does the loudness of your tinnitus change on its own?

Tinnitus loudness may seem to change due to:

- Exposure to certain sounds
- Eating certain foods
- Being under extreme stress
- Being sleep deprived
- New medications or changes in dosage
- Changes in daily acoustic environment.

The patient's answer to this question should not reflect these types of events. The purpose of the question is to determine whether the tinnitus fluctuates in loudness *on its own*, and if so, how often. "On its own" thus refers to naturally occurring changes in tinnitus loudness, that is, there is no external factor that precipitates the change.

Spontaneous changes in loudness can be associated with the tinnitus being more or less bothersome, that is, when the tinnitus is louder it tends to be more intrusive and annoying; when it is softer it might not be noticed as much. With PTM, patients are taught how to manage situations when their tinnitus is bothersome. With spontaneous changes in tinnitus loudness, these bothersome situations might be contingent on the loudness of the tinnitus.

Question 2: Do sounds ever change the loudness of your tinnitus? What kinds of sounds make your tinnitus louder? When sound makes your tinnitus louder, how long does the change last?

Patients occasionally report that exposure to certain sounds causes an increase in the loudness of their tinnitus (P. J. Jastreboff & Hazell, 2004). Dangerously loud sounds would be expected to cause this effect. One of the response options is "very loud sounds." If this is the patient's response, then exacerbation of tinnitus by sound most likely would be a normal effect and the patient should be counseled regarding hearing conservation. The intent of the question, however, is whether sounds at nondamaging levels cause the tinnitus to increase in loudness. If this is experienced, then the effect usually lasts minutes or hours. Of most concern is whether the effect lasts until at least the next day.

It may be helpful for patients who experience a prolonged tinnitus-exacerbation effect due to sound to carry earplugs so as to remain prepared for unavoidable situations that could trigger the exacerbation. Custom-fit high-fidelity/musicians earplugs usually are considered comfortable and they minimize distortion of sound. Patients must be cautioned, however, to *avoid overuse* of earplugs that could further increase their sensitivity to sound (Formby et al., 2002). Patients who experience prolonged exacerbation of tinnitus from sound also may require intervention for hyperacusis (see Chapter 6).

Question 3: How does your tinnitus affect you (not including trouble hearing or understanding speech)?

This question supplements the questions from Section A of the THS, which mentions specific life situations that commonly are affected by tinnitus. It is important to ask this open-ended question so that patients identify, without any prompting, the most bothersome aspects of their tinnitus. As always, it is important to ensure that patients do not confuse their tinnitus complaints with "trouble hearing or understanding speech." A patient's answer to Question 3 should indicate the primary complaint(s) that will be targeted by the intervention.

Question 4: Please tell me about everything you tried for your tinnitus prior to PTM. For each effort, what were you hoping would happen, and what actually did happen?

This question includes a note to the clinician, which helps to clarify the intent of asking the question:

Clinician: Sometimes a pattern will emerge showing that the patient has made repeated (unsuccessful) attempts to make the tinnitus quieter, resulting in frustration and distress. If this is the case, try to ensure that the patient begins to see this pattern more clearly.

The discussion elicited by this question is useful to both the clinician and patient as they identify everything the patient has attempted for tinnitus management and the effectiveness of each effort. In the process, it may become evident that the patient made repeated attempts to *quiet* the tinnitus and that each unsuccessful effort compounded the distress. The clinician should help the patient recognize if this has been the pattern of previous attempts to manage tinnitus. If so, then the clinician should clarify that the goal of intervention with PTM never is to change the tinnitus, and to explain the rationale for this approach. Throughout the course of PTM a patient might unintentionally slip back into the pattern of trying to change the tinnitus; if the clinician understands the patient's history of attempts to change the tinnitus and the results of those attempts, then the clinician can gently remind the patient of that unsatisfactory history.

Question 5: Please tell me about the sounds you have used to manage your reactions to tinnitus since starting PTM. For each sound you tried, what were you hoping would happen, and what actually did happen?

As for Question 4, this question includes a note to the clinician to clarify the question's intent:

Clinician: if the patient has the Sound Plan Worksheets that were used during Level 3, these can be used to guide this interaction. It also is important to reinforce the idea that with PTM the goal is not to change the tinnitus, but rather to change how one feels.

The intent of this question is to determine the patient's impressions regarding his or her experiences using therapeutic sound with PTM. It is helpful if any Sound Plan Worksheets (see Appendix N) used by the patient are available for discussion. The clinician should note any misunderstandings or unrealistic expectations regarding the use of sound and reinstruct the patient as necessary to ensure that expectations are realistic. It also is helpful for the clinician to identify any successes experienced by the patient so that they can be pointed out and built upon if the patient continues with PTM.

Question 6: If we decide to move ahead with one-on-one support, then we will be making plans for using sound to manage your reactions to tinnitus. It will be helpful to have a list of sound-producing devices that you have available to you. Which of the following devices do you own?

As for Questions 4 and 5, a note to the clinician is included to clarify the question's intent:

Clinician: For each type of device listed below that the patient owns, provide additional details. For instance, if patients report they own a radio, ask: how many radios, if any of them are portable, and if not portable where it is located. For each device the patient owns, ask how it currently is being used relative to tinnitus management.

Patients sometimes overlook sources of sound that they already own that can be used to manage their reactions to tinnitus. Answering this question creates a fairly detailed list of all of these resources available to the patient. The list can be referred to whenever a Sound Plan Worksheet is created or modified. All of the items on the list should be those that the patient already owns or has access to. Creating this list also can lead to discussion concerning other types of sound-producing devices that might be helpful for future sound plans.

Psychoacoustic Assessment of Tinnitus

Psychoacoustic assessment of tinnitus generally is not recommended within the framework of PTM.

This may seem surprising, so the rationale for this recommendation is provided below.

A tinnitus psychoacoustic assessment typically includes tinnitus loudness and pitch matching, finding the minimum masking level (MML) using broadband noise (BBN), and testing for residual inhibition (RI). Tinnitus loudness and pitch matching involves procedures designed to identify a pure tone or band of noise that matches as closely as possible the pitch and loudness of the tinnitus. MML testing consists of finding the level of BBN required to completely cover, or mask the tinnitus. RI refers to the phenomenon that tinnitus can be temporarily reduced or terminated following certain acoustic stimulation.

When these tests are performed, patients are asked to attend closely to their tinnitus and to the effects of different sounds on the tinnitus. Asking patients to pay close attention to the sound of their tinnitus is at cross purposes with the therapeutic goals of PTM. With PTM, patients are required to attend to how they feel, rather than to the sound of their tinnitus. Making the transition to attending to how they feel and their *reactions* to tinnitus rather than to the sound of tinnitus is difficult for many patients, but very important. It is important because patients usually cannot satisfactorily change the sound of their tinnitus, but they usually can change how they feel. Furthermore, for PTM, results of tinnitus psychoacoustic testing generally are not helpful for diagnostic purposes, for guiding intervention, or for assessing outcomes of intervention.

An argument sometimes made for performing these tests is that results of pitch matching can be useful when adjusting the frequency output of an ear-level sound generator. The hope is that providing more sound in the frequency range corresponding with the tinnitus pitch will result in improved masking of tinnitus. Such efforts are irrelevant and possibly counterproductive with respect to using therapeutic sound with PTM. For example, sound from an ear-level sound generator would be used either as background sound or soothing sound (see Chapter 7). If used as background sound, then achieving masking is of no consequence—the purpose of background sound is to reduce contrast between tinnitus and a quiet environment. If used as soothing sound, then the audiologist should adjust the frequency output of the sound generator to produce a soothing effect regardless of the effect on the tinnitus itself. Patients commonly report that some sounds are soothing or relaxing even if they have no effect on the tinnitus percept. Conversely, some patients report that sounds that mask their tinnitus are unacceptably loud, or are as unpleasant as the tinnitus itself. Therefore, for PTM, focusing on masking tinnitus by emphasizing sound in the frequency range that corresponds with the pitch match can hinder efforts to identify sounds that are soothing to the patient.

Another argument sometimes made is that results of MML testing can be useful in predicting which patients are likely to benefit from the use of ear-level noise/sound generators (alone or in combination with a hearing aid). The rationale behind this argument is that patients who require high levels of BBN to mask their tinnitus are more likely to require unacceptably high levels of sound from a sound generator to adequately mask their tinnitus. As explained above, masking tinnitus is not the goal of using sound with PTM. (Masking may occur, however, in the process of using sound for another therapeutic purpose.) With PTM, sound from an ear-level sound generator is used either as soothing sound or background sound—neither of which involves masking of tinnitus. Therefore, predicting that a patient is unlikely to benefit from the use of ear-level sound generators because of high MMLs may falsely lower expectations of benefit and could actually prevent a patient from discovering that using a sound generator can be helpful for providing soothing or background sound even if there is no effect on the sound of the tinnitus itself.

For these reasons tinnitus psychoacoustic testing is not recommended as part of the Level 4 Interdisciplinary Evaluation. However, PTM should be considered a framework within which flexibility is allowed (and even encouraged) to best meet the needs of individual clinical programs. Detailed instructions for tinnitus psychoacoustic testing have been published elsewhere (J. A. Henry, 2004; J. A. Henry, Zaugg, & Schechter, 2005a) for clinicians who wish to include it in their clinical protocol.

In-Clinic Trials of Ear-Level Instruments (optional procedures)

Patients who reach Level 4 have undergone a successive "filtering" process that provides reasonable assurance that their problem with tinnitus warrants individualized clinical attention. These patients generally require much more assistance than has been available to them up to this point. They also typically are motivated to try new strategies that might be helpful in managing their reactions to tinnitus.

At Level 4, all types of ear-level sound generators and combination instruments (and hearing aids) are viable options for intervention. (Please refer to the Flowchart for Assessment and Fitting of Ear-level Instruments—Appendix I). The normal protocol is to fit only hearing aids at Level 2. However, as noted in Chapter 5, new models of combination instruments provide full-feature hearing aids. These combination instruments can be fitted at Level 2, and, if so, then we would recommend that the noise generator portion be turned off until the patient has received the audiologic counseling that is provided at Level 3.

If results of the Tinnitus and Hearing Survey (see Appendix D), supplemented with the Tinnitus Interview (see Appendix R) suggest that a patient is a candidate for Level 5 Individualized Support from an audiologist, then—if the patient is amenable—it is appropriate to conduct in-clinic trials of ear-level instruments. It is important to perform *in-clinic* trials because it often is difficult to predict how a patient's tinnitus (and reactions to tinnitus) will be affected by amplification, sound from an ear-level sound generator, or a combination of amplification plus sound generator. In-clinic trial use of ear-level instruments allows patients to make realistic, experience-based decisions about the potential effectiveness of the devices. It should be explained to patients that the purpose of the in-clinic trials is to evaluate the potential usefulness of the devices for ongoing management of reactions to tinnitus. Results of the trials are used to determine collaboratively if ear-level instruments will be provided before beginning Level 5 Individualized Support.

Three Categories of Patients at Level 4

Categorizing patients with respect to their candidacy for hearing aids is essential prior to the Level 4 in-clinic trials of ear-level instruments. Different instruments are demonstrated depending on the patient's category. Categories include: (a) obvious hearing aid candidate; (b) borderline hearing aid candidate; and (c) not a hearing aid candidate.

"Obvious hearing aid candidates" are patients who have hearing loss to such a degree that: (a) amplification would most likely ameliorate their communicative and other hearing problems; and (b) they are motivated to wear hearing aids. With PTM, hearing aids typically are fit at Level 2 (see Appendix I). Therefore, at Level 4, most obvious hearing aid candidates will already be wearing hearing aids.

"Borderline hearing aid candidates" typically report "occasional hearing problems." These patients tend to have mild to moderate sloping high-frequency sensorineural hearing loss. To be considered a borderline hearing aid candidate, patients must be motivated to wear hearing aids (for management of tinnitus and/or to improve hearing).

Which Ear-Level Instruments Should Be Demonstrated for Each Patient Category?

For "obvious" and "borderline" hearing aid candidates, in-clinic trials with hearing aids and combination instruments are conducted. (If the patient already is a hearing aid user, then an in-clinic trial using the patient's current hearing aids should be performed.) Borderline hearing aid candidates also should be evaluated for noise generators.

For patients who are not hearing aid candidates, normally only in-clinic trials with noise generators should be conducted. However, some patients with essentially normal hearing will benefit from hearing aids that are optimized for patients with tinnitus (described later).

Special Forms to Guide In-Clinic Trials of Ear-Level Instruments

A series of four forms has been developed for use as guides to selecting ear-level instruments at the Level 4 Interdisciplinary Evaluation. These forms include:

- Guide to Trial Use of Ear-Level Instruments (Appendix V)
- In-Clinic Trial Use of Hearing Aids (Appendix W)
- In-Clinic Trial Use of Combination Instruments (Appendix X)
- In-Clinic Trial Use of Noise Generators (Appendix Y)

The first form (Guide to Trial Use of Ear-Level Instruments—Appendix V) gives an overview of which ear-level instruments should be tried in the clinic for patients who are:

- Obvious hearing aid candidates
- Borderline hearing aid candidates
- Not hearing aid candidates.

This form also contains a guide to discussing with patients results of the trials and collaboratively making decisions regarding the use of ear-level instruments during Level 5 Individualized Support. The other forms (In-Clinic Trial Use of Hearing Aids—Appendix W; In-Clinic Trial Use of Combination Instruments—Appendix X; In-Clinic Trial Use of Noise Generators—Appendix Y) provide detailed instructions for conducting the in-clinic trials. These forms also are used to record patient responses to each trial performed.

Clinic Inventory of Trial Ear-Level Instruments

A variety of ear-level instruments should be available to conduct in-clinic trials with patients. Because of potential sanitization concerns, in-the-ear (ITE) instruments are not recommended—only behind-the-ear (BTE) instruments with temporary disposable earmolds are used for in-clinic trial use. Certain supplies also should be on hand, such as temporary earmolds (in a variety of sizes with variable venting), vent plugs, and temporary feedback wraps.

Minimum Inventory of Ear-Level Instruments for In-Clinic Trial Use

The minimum inventory of ear-level instruments would be a single pair of BTE combination instruments (with disposable earmolds). If possible, the instruments should have an adjustable frequency response for both the amplifier and the noise generator. If trial instruments are limited to one set of BTE combination instruments, then these instruments can be used to demonstrate the potential benefit from:

Noise Generators Alone. BTE combination instruments can be used to demonstrate the benefit obtained from using ear-level noise generators (the hearing aid portion is turned off).

Hearing Aids Alone. BTE combination instruments can be used to demonstrate the benefit obtained from using hearing aids (the noise generator portion is turned off). The drawback is that the hearing aid portion of a combination instrument may be less flexible, less sophisticated, and have fewer features than a traditional hearing aid. Increasingly, new models of combination instruments do not sacrifice hearing aid features, so these potential drawbacks are becoming less of a concern.

Combined Noise Generator and Hearing Aid. BTE combination instruments can be used to demonstrate the potential benefit from the simultaneous use of a noise generator and hearing aid (both are turned on at the same time).

Ideal Inventory of Ear-Level Instruments for In-Clinic Trial Use

The ideal inventory of stock ear-level instruments would include noise generators, combination instruments, and hearing aids. There should be a pair of each type of device to allow binaural trial fittings of each. If possible, more than one model/make of noise generator and combination instrument should be available to demonstrate the different choices. Hearing aids that serve a wide fitting range should be on hand.

Personal listening devices and stationary devices such as tabletop sound conditioners, pillow speakers, and MP3 players loaded with interesting, soothing, and background sounds also should be available for patients to try as alternative therapeutic uses of sound if ear-level instruments are not advised or desired.

Maintaining Continuity Between Level 3 Counseling and In-Clinic Trials

During the Level 3 Group Education workshops, patients learn about the three types of sound (soothing, background, interesting) that can be used to manage reactions to tinnitus (see Chapter 7). For the in-clinic trials to be most meaningful, patients need to be informed that the instruments can be used to provide an immediate sense of relief (soothing sound), to provide a background of sound to reduce the tinnitus/background contrast, and to improve access to interesting sound.

Need for Follow-Up If Patients Receive Ear-Level Instruments

Use of ear-level instruments for tinnitus requires ongoing support (Level 5 Individualized Support) from an audiologist, including continued development and assessment of strategies for using sound most effectively. This process is facilitated by using the Sound Plan Worksheet (see Appendix N), which should be reviewed at every appointment. Individualized support typically involves two to five visits over a period of up to 6 months. A patient who receives special ear-level devices during Level 4 should attend at least two Level 5 appointments.

Fitting Appointment

If ear-level instruments were ordered for the patient, then they are fitted prior to the initial Level 5 appointment. However, the fitting appointment can be combined with the initial Level 5 appointment (which makes for a very long appointment).

Summary of Ear-Level Instruments for PTM

Appropriate use of sound can be critically important for managing reactions to tinnitus. There are numerous options for using sound with ear-level instruments. Each option must be considered for the individual patient. A systematic approach is required to determine the best combination of instruments and sounds. The patient makes the final decision, and the clinician facilitates the decision making process and provides a selection of sounds and instruments.

Criteria for Patients to Progress to Level 5 Individualized Support

Following completion of the Level 4 Interdisciplinary Evaluation for a patient, ideally the psychologist, audiologist, and patient decide collaboratively if the patient will initiate Level 5 Individualized Support with the psychologist and/or audiologist. Patients must meet the following criteria to be considered for Level 5 Individualized Support:

- Levels 1 to 4 of PTM have not adequately addressed their tinnitus concerns.
- They have been evaluated and referred as appropriate for care in other clinics.
- They understand the nature of the PTM services available from the psychologist and audiologist (including device options and potential duration of intervention).
- They are motivated and capable of participating in the activities proposed by the psychologist and/or audiologist.

If Level 5 Individualized Support is initiated with both the psychologist and audiologist, it is best if the clinicians remain in regular contact regarding the patient's progress within each of the disciplines.

9

Level 5 Individualized Support

PTM

Progressive Tinnitus Management

Individualized support is needed by relatively few patients. Level 5 Individualized Support involves use of the same principles of using sound and coping techniques to manage tinnitus that are presented in Level 3 Group Education. However, at Level 5 some patients use ear-level noise/sound generators or combination instruments, and the education and support is provided in a one-on-one format with more intense and individualized assistance. Also, Level 5 counseling is less structured and allows for flexibility in what is covered during the sessions. The individual counseling should reinforce the Level 3 principles, but the clinician has latitude to modify or expand on the counseling information as needed. Level 5 intervention normally requires up to six months of repeated appointments with an audiologist and/or a mental health provider.

Level 5 Standard Protocol for Audiologists

Level 5 Appointments

At each Level 5 appointment with an audiologist: (a) the functioning and proper use of ear-level instruments is verified (if applicable); and (b) one-on-one PTM counseling is conducted—focusing on updating the Sound Plan Worksheet (see Appendix N) to ensure that the patient is optimizing the use of therapeutic sound to address tinnitus-problem situations. If the clinician feels that it is necessary, the patient's progress is evaluated, and current needs are assessed using any of the questionnaires that were administered at the Level 4 evaluation, including the Tinnitus Handicap Inventory (see Appendix F),

Tinnitus and Hearing Survey (see Appendix D), Hearing Handicap Inventory (see Appendix G), and the Tinnitus Interview (see Appendix R). If the Tinnitus Interview is used, then it is best to select individual questions that are relevant to the patient's complaints rather than administering the entire interview. Audiometric testing is repeated only if the patient reports a significant auditory change.

Schedule of Appointments

Following the initial Level 5 appointment, return counseling appointments normally are scheduled at 1, 2, 4, and 6 months.

Why Are Return Appointments Important?

Return appointments are an essential, but often neglected, aspect of ongoing management for patients who have a severe problem with tinnitus. It is unreasonable to expect these patients to accomplish all management objectives without the guidance and support of a tinnitus specialist. Consequently, they require repeated appointments on a prescribed schedule until their problem is sufficiently resolved and/or they are capable of performing self-management effectively.

From a health education perspective, patients need to return for repeated counseling because they recall only about half of the information, and some of the health information is remembered incorrectly (Margolis, 2004; Shapiro, Boggs, Melamed, & Graham-Pole, 1992). It also has been reported that patients immediately forget as much as 80% of the information (Kessels, 2003).

Repeated appointments are required for all Level 5 patients to ensure that they are using their ear-level devices properly and that they remember the key points of counseling (J. A. Henry, Trune et al., 2007a; P. J. Jastreboff & Hazell, 2004). Return visits also are necessary to ensure that patients are (a) implementing their individualized sound plans developed at previous visits, and modifying the plans to optimize their efficacy; and (b) using the specific coping skills that are taught by the mental health provider. Compliance with a schedule of periodic appointments optimizes the potential to achieve successful results.

Adherence to the Appointment Schedule

Adherence to the recommended schedule requires motivation and commitment on the part of the patient. Normally, only patients with the most problematic tinnitus are so inclined. Patients who live at a distance may not be able to return to the clinic as often as advised. These patients should at least be counseled via telephone, using the self-help workbook *How to Manage Your Tinnitus: A Step-by-Step Workbook* (J. A. Henry et al., 2010a) as a general guide to implementing self-help strategies.

Six-Month Appointment

The appointment at six months is the final appointment for most patients receiving Level 5 services. If this is the final appointment, then the same procedures are conducted as for the standard protocol that is recommended for all of the Level 5 appointments (see Level 5 Appointments above). In addition, the Tinnitus Handicap Inventory (see Appendix F) and the Tinnitus and Hearing Survey (see Appendix D) should be administered and results compared to previous responses to evaluate the patient's progress through all levels of PTM. If problems were reported on the Tinnitus Interview (see Appendix R), then it would be important to repeat any pertinent questions from the interview.

Exceptions to the Level 5 Standard Protocol for Audiologists

Final Appointment

The patient's final Level 5 appointment may be earlier or later than six-months. Regardless of when the final appointment takes place, the procedures described above for the six-month appointment should be performed during the final appointment.

Making the Decision to End Intervention Before or After Six Months

The decision to end intervention should be made jointly between the clinician and patient. Ideally, this decision would be corroborated by the patient's responses to outcome questions on the Tinnitus Handicap Inventory (THI) (see Appendix F) and Tinnitus and Hearing Survey (see Appendix D) (although such corroboration is not essential). As a reference, it has been reported that a 20-point reduction in the THI index score reflects "clinically significant improvement" (C. W. Newman & Sandridge, 2004). When intervention is complete, patients should be advised to telephone the clinician whenever questions or issues arise, and to request special appointments if needed.

Extending Intervention Beyond Six Months

If the patient requires intervention beyond six months, then the progress made to this point should be reviewed with the patient along with discussion of the potential benefit of further intervention. Multiple issues can be discussed as potentially contributing to a lack of sufficient progress:

- The patient's tinnitus problem was so severe that more time and support are needed for the patient to be able to adequately self-manage reactions to tinnitus.
- Effective sound plans (using the Sound Plan Worksheet—Appendix N) have not yet been identified.
- The patient (for any reason) has not implemented the sound plan(s) from the Sound Plan Worksheet.
- A psychological component has not been properly managed through help from a mental health professional.

Every possible contributing factor should be explored, and referrals to other services may be indicated more strongly at this point. If, after thorough review with the patient, there is agreement that further intervention may be helpful, then Level 5 appointments can be extended beyond six months. It is critical for these patients to know that further services are accessible and available if needed.

Telephone Counseling

Patients may not be able to attend the recommended series of return appointments because they live at a distance or for other reasons. These patients can be counseled adequately over the telephone if they have the self-help workbook (J. A. Henry et al., 2010a) to refer to during the counseling.

Self-Help Workbook

At the initial Level 5 appointment, patients should be asked if they have a copy of the workbook (*How to Manage Your Tinnitus: A Step-by-Step Guide,* J. A. Henry et al., 2010a), which normally is dispensed at the beginning of Level 3 Group Education. If not, then a new copy should be provided. The workbook should be reviewed with the patient and portions of the workbook that are most applicable should be discussed. Patients should be aware that the key PTM counseling principles are described in the workbook, along with step-by-step instructions for developing plans to manage their tinnitus problem using both therapeutic sound and coping techniques. They should be encouraged to read the workbook and adhere to its recommendations.

PTM Level 5 Counseling

The education provided by audiologists to patients at all levels of PTM is designed primarily to help patients develop, and experience success using, self-management strategies that address the situations when their tinnitus is most problematic (using the Sound Plan Worksheet—Appendix N). The main difference at Level 5 is the one-on-one setting that facilitates direct interaction between patient and clinician. Some patients do better by receiving ongoing individualized attention from a caring and knowledgeable clinician. Some patients also need the opportunity to resolve any questions or concerns about their tinnitus in a private setting where they can express feelings and concerns that they might not have been comfortable discussing in a group setting.

A patient counseling guide (*Progressive Tinnitus Management: Counseling Guide*, J. A. Henry et al., 2010b) is used during the Level 5 appointments. The counseling guide is used like a flip chart, but laid flat on a table between clinician and patient. When the book is open, one side faces the clinician and the other side faces the patient. The clinician's pages contain bulleted counseling points, and the patient's pages show simplified bulleted points and illustrative graphics. The counseling guide was designed to be used primarily by audiologists. A similar guide is in development that will be intended primarily for use by mental health providers.

The Level 5 patient counseling guide includes three sections: an introductory section, follow-up section, and supplemental sound tolerance (hyperacusis) section. The first two sections correspond with the Level 3 PowerPoint presentations (*Managing Your Tinnitus: What to Do and How to Do It*) that are included on the CD in the back of this handbook. Using the counseling guide, most patients at Level 5 will start with the follow-up section (because the material covered in the introductory section was already covered during Level 3 Group Education). The introductory section normally is used only with patients who have not completed Level 3. The introductory section, however, serves as a resource for fundamental PTM counseling information that can be accessed as needed during counseling sessions.

Demonstrating Personal Listening Devices and Stationary Devices

Appropriate use of augmentative sound can be very effective for helping to manage reactions to tinnitus. Unless the various personal listening devices and stationary devices are demonstrated in the clinic, however, patients may not appreciate their full value. There is no formal protocol for demonstrating these devices—they simply should be available in the clinic and demonstrated as appropriate during the Level 5 appointments.

Level 5 CBT

The Level 4 Interdisciplinary Evaluation informs the intervention provided by a mental health provider at Level 5. The mental health services at Level 5 involve a review of the CBT coping techniques taught during Level 3 Group Education (and included in the self-help workbook that is provided to patients at Level 3) and an individualized examination of patients' unique achievements and challenges so far during PTM. Further integrating coping skills by attending to challenges patients face when implementing the skills allows themes to emerge. Patients learn more about setting and achieving goals with behavioral modification by tracking their progress using clearly defined measures of change. For example, if a patient is having difficulty managing stress, charting stress on a scale from 0 to 10 is an effective way to quantify the patient's response to stress and observe change as a result of modification in behavior. During Level 5, patients learn how to accept their individual strengths and weaknesses while gaining a sense of control in the event that change is realistic and obtainable.

In order to provide CBT, clinicians must be trained by another professional experienced in this modality of psychotherapy. Mental health clinicians may or may not have received this training, thus the involvement of mental health at this level will depend on the availability of CBT-trained mental health providers. A mental health provider who is experienced in providing CBT is skilled in explaining the process of CBT to patients, possesses skill in conceptualizing underlying themes that arise for individuals, and assists patients in developing their skills to problem solve. Such clinicians refer to themselves as "psychotherapists," which is a title regulated by state licensing boards based on qualifications and training. A psychotherapist has received years of training and supervision on establishing a good working relationship with patients (also known as rapport). Psychotherapists adhere to a code of ethics and guide patients through the therapeutic intervention. Psychotherapists who specifically provide CBT understand the importance of behavioral and cognitive theories of the intervention. They assist the patients in learning ways to evaluate and change their thoughts and behaviors.

During Level 5 CBT, psychotherapists help patients understand their tinnitus as it relates to the entire mind-body system. Often, tinnitus is accompanied by symptoms of depression such as increased or decreased appetite, problems falling or staying asleep, and decreased pleasure when doing activities that once were pleasurable, among other symptoms. By simultaneously addressing a patient's reactions to tinnitus and depressive symptoms, the patient recognizes the importance of addressing both the mind's reactions to physical symptoms, and the physical symptoms that might influence emotions.

Occasionally, patients place more emphasis on the problem of tinnitus than on other more difficult emotional problems, such as unresolved trauma. Perhaps because tinnitus adds to frustration that already exists for some patients who struggle when negative emotions arise or because tinnitus is something that can be described physically, learning ways to cope with tinnitus may be how patients prefer to begin looking at the way they cope with stress, emotions, and problems in general. Nonetheless, several patients during one of our studies (see Chapter 2, Fifth Study) who began using CBT to cope with tinnitus realized that their tinnitus was just one problem among many in their lives. CBT for tinnitus for these particular patients offers an introduction to positive thoughts, behaviors, and attitudes in what might be perceived as a less formidable environment than what would be required to address the "other problems." Such patients are then primed to use these coping skills in other areas of their lives. Level 5 CBT gives patients the opportunity to start using the skills of CBT on a concrete, diagnosable, physical problem (tinnitus) from which they can apply the skills to more global emotional problems and behaviors.

Case Study: Sam

Sam has received ongoing Level 5 Individualized Support fom an audiologist and psychologist for three months. He reports that his combination instruments have been helpful, but lately has been finding that he has to turn up the noise generator higher and higher to completely "mask out" the tinnitus. He also reports that once he has set the noise generator to a high level, sometimes the tinnitus returns after several minutes. He also feels like he is carrying around his own portable noisy environment and believes he cannot hear as well when the noise is on.

Sam needs to be reminded that the goal of using sound is never to mask the tinnitus. The three types of sound (soothing, interesting, and background) should be reviewed. It should be clarified that the sound generator portion of the combination instrument can be used as soothing sound or background sound, neither of which requires masking. It may also be helpful to point out that the hearing aid portion of the device can make it easier for him to understand interesting sounds—like speech. It also can be explained that when hearing is the predominant need, he can turn the noise to either a very soft level or turn it off completely.

The audiologist should summarize the contents of the meeting with Sam and make it available to the psychologist providing Level 5 support to ensure that the psychologist is aware of Sam's difficulties with using sound.

Beyond Level 5 Individualized Support

If a patient does not make satisfactory progress after about six months of Level 5 Individualized Support, then a different approach can be considered. Options for extended intervention at Level 5 include further PTM audiologic counseling (modified as necessary), further CBT counseling (including the addition of different components of CBT that may not have been covered to this point), tinnitus masking, tinnitus retraining therapy, and neuromonics tinnitus treatment. There is no definitive evidence that any one of these behavioral methods is more effective than any other.

Cognitive-Behavioral Therapy

The objectives of CBT are to identify negative behaviors, beliefs, and reactions in patients and to assist them in substituting appropriate and positive reactions (see Chapter 7). CBT initially was used as an effective treatment for depression and anxiety. A standard CBT protocol as adapted for tinnitus involves up to ten sessions. These sessions can be conducted with individual patients or with groups of patients.

CBT normally is performed by mental health providers. It can, however, be administered by other health care providers who have received the proper training. Training to conduct CBT for tinnitus is not offered on any routine basis for nonmental health clinicians, but must be obtained from a professional who has this expertise. Books are available that describe CBT clinical procedures in detail (J. L. Henry & P. H. Wilson, 1998, 2002).

Tinnitus Masking

The method of tinnitus masking (TM) became available as a clinical technique in the late 1970s (Vernon, 1977). It was popular through the 1980s and continues to be used (Schechter & J. A. Henry, 2002). The main objective of TM is to use broadband noise to provide a sense of relief from tension or stress caused by tinnitus. Because of the label "masking," however, the main objective has commonly been misunderstood to be to cover up or "mask" the tinnitus (J. A. Henry, Schechter, et al., 2002). Maximizing a sense of relief is accomplished with complete masking for some people, partial masking for others, and sometimes even with no masking effect (J. A. Henry, Rheinsburg, & Zaugg, 2004).

TM patients normally are fitted with ear-level instruments ("maskers") that present wide-band noise to the ears. Patients are instructed to adjust the noise to the level that provides the greatest sense of relief. With respect to the PTM combinations of sound (see Figure 7-1), TM is an example of *using environmental sound as soothing sound*. Patients also are advised to use various sound-producing devices to achieve relief, including CDs, tabletop fountains, sound machines, sound pillows, and so forth. Counseling is used with TM, but the use of therapeutic sound to induce a sense of relief is the primary mode of intervention. There is no training program available for TM. Clinicians must learn TM on their own or be trained by an individual who has expertise in this method.

Tinnitus Retraining Therapy

The method of tinnitus retraining therapy (TRT) has two basic components: educational ("directive") counseling and "sound therapy" (J. A. Henry, Trune, et al., 2007a, 2007b; P. J. Jastreboff & Hazell, 2004). Unlike TM, the use of therapeutic sound with TRT is not meant to give a sense of relief (J. A. Henry, Schechter, et al., 2002). With TRT the patient should hear the tinnitus clearly, but with constant sound in the background. The background sound reduces the contrast between the tinnitus and the quiet environment, thus making the tinnitus less likely to attract attention (passive attention diversion). Patients are supposed to use sound in this way every day to eventually achieve habituation, that is, reduction or elimination of tinnitus reactions and perception.

Evaluation of patients for TRT results in their placement into one of five categories: 0, 1, 2, 3, and 4. Patients in all categories are counseled to "enrich their sound environment" at all times with soft, pleasant, or neutral background sound. Category 0 patients have tinnitus that is not severe enough to warrant the use of ear-level devices, thus they receive TRT counseling only. Category 1 patients are severely bothered by their tinnitus, and ear-level instruments (sound generators, combination instruments, or hearing aids) are advised for use each day for at least one year. With respect to the PTM combinations of sound (see Figure 7–1), the use of broadband noise with TRT is an example of *using environmental sound as background sound*.

Category 2 patients also have a severe tinnitus problem, but in addition they have hearing loss requiring amplification. These patients are fitted with hearing aids or combination instruments, and sound therapy is conducted as for Category 1 patients. Patients in Category 3 require primary management for hyperacusis, which involves special desensitization procedures using sound to increase tolerance levels (J. A. Henry, Trune, et al., 2007a, 2007b). Category 4 refers to patients whose tinnitus is exacerbated by exposure to certain sounds. These latter patients require judicious use of sound to systematically reduce their reactions to sound.

The originators of this method contend that it is necessary to attend their training courses in order to properly conduct TRT. However, books are available that describe TRT clinical procedures in detail, and numerous clinicians who are trained and experienced in conducting TRT may be available to provide training and clinical supervision.

Neuromonics Tinnitus Treatment

Neuromonics tinnitus treatment (NTT) is unique among tinnitus therapies in that providers who offer this technique work directly with a company to receive all training, materials, therapeutic devices, and support. After a provider has received training, company representatives attend the provider's first appointments with patients to ensure that all clinical procedures are conducted according to the prescribed protocol. The method cannot be implemented without the company's endorsement and support.

Intervention with NTT involves six months or more of using a proprietary, wearable listening device 2 to 3 hours per day (P. B. Davis, 2006). The device is similar to an MP3 player and plays baroque and new age music that is specially selected for having relaxation-inducing qualities. For each patient, the device is customized by the company so that the sound output is adjusted (equalized) for any hearing loss. The device is used to implement desensitization to the tinnitus in two stages as the prescribed protocol. During the first two months of treatment (stage 1) wide-band noise ("shower sound") is added to the music. The objective of stage 1 is to attain a sense of relief and control over the tinnitus—generally to reduce anxiety. Relative to the combinations of sound as described for PTM (see Figure 7–1), the use of sound during stage 1 of NTT is an example of *using a combination of music and environmental sound as soothing sound*. During the next four months (stage 2) the wide-band noise is removed from the audio signal. Patients are instructed to gradually reduce the volume of the music. The objective of stage 2 is essentially the same as for TRT: less awareness of, and less reaction to, the tinnitus. The use of sound during stage 2 of NTT is an example of *using music as soothing sound*, transitioning to *using music as background sound* (see Figure 7–1) prior to discontinuing daily use of the device.

Conclusion

All audiologists routinely encounter patients who complain of tinnitus. Different methods of intervention for tinnitus have been available to audiologists for years. However, relatively few audiologists have received adequate training in providing clinical services for tinnitus. Audiologists need the skills to evaluate patients and provide the needed level of care. The method of PTM is a definable program of care that is based primarily on goal-oriented counseling of various uses of sound for managing reactions to tinnitus, and the provision of specific coping skills fundamental to CBT.

Standardized clinical guidelines for managing reactions to tinnitus are unlikely to be established in the near future for audiologists. Training in tinnitus clinical services is highly variable among audiology graduate programs (J. A. Henry, Zaugg, et al., 2005a). Any training that exists reflects biases, which is understandable because research does not conclusively support any one form of management. There are four broad areas that require consensus to achieve standardization. These include: (a) defined clinical procedures; (b) research evidence to support clinical procedures; (c) audiology graduate training; and (d) patient educational programs. PTM establishes basic procedures that can be used by audiologists until more formal standardized techniques are developed and validated.

The effectiveness of intervention with PTM depends on the effectiveness of the education that is provided to patients. It is essential that evidence-based methods of patient education are utilized. Previously, we have reviewed a variety of learning theories that have particular relevance to PTM

(J. A. Henry, Zaugg, Myers, Kendall, et al., 2009). This review shows that PTM adheres to a number of principles that have been demonstrated to optimize effective patient learning of skills for self-management of health.

We recognize that counseling for facilitating health behavior change presents challenges that can result in frustration for patients and clinicians alike (Rollnick, Mason, & Butler, 1999). Behavioral changes do not come easily, especially when the target behaviors and their underlying cognitions are long-standing, sometimes even lifelong habits. However, counseling with PTM is a patient-centered method that addresses the uniqueness of each patient and his or her particular tinnitus-problem profile. This patient-centered approach has been shown to greatly enhance individual motivation for making adaptive changes for improving health (Stewart et al., 2000). In PTM, patients participate in the process of defining the problem and identifying specific behavior changes for managing the problem. Each patient becomes an active participant in making decisions and ultimately is in charge of making lifestyle adjustments to mitigate his or her own tinnitus problem. Understanding that the patient is an expert in his or her own life circumstances, problems, resources, and abilities is the key that enables this collaborative tinnitus self-management approach to succeed.

References

PTM

Progressive Tinnitus Management

Axelsson, A., & Barrenas, M. -L. (1992). Tinnitus in noise-induced hearing loss. In A. L. Dancer, D. Henderson, R. J. Salvi & R. P. Hamnernik (Eds.), *Noise-induced hearing loss* (pp. 269–276). St. Louis, MO: Mosby-Year Book.

Axelsson, A., & Ringdahl, A. (1989). Tinnitus: A study of its prevalence and characteristics. *British Journal of Audiology, 23*, 53–62.

Baguley, D. M. (2002). Mechanisms of tinnitus. *British Medical Bulletin, 63*, 195–212.

Baker, D. W., Parker, R. M., Williams, M. V., Clark, W. S., & Nurss, J. (1997). The relationship of patient reading ability to self-reported health and use of health services. *American Journal of Public Health, 87*(6), 1027–1030.

Bandura, A. (1977). Self-efficacy: Toward a unifying theory of behavioral change. *Psychological Review, 84*(2), 191–215.

Bartnik, G., Fabijanska, A., & Rogowski, M. (2001). Effects of tinnitus retraining therapy (TRT) for patients with tinnitus and subjective hearing loss versus tinnitus only. *Scandinavian Audiology Supplement, 52*, 206–208.

Battaglia, A., Burchette, R., & Cueva, R. (2008). Combination therapy (intratympanic dexamethasone + high-dose prednisone taper) for the treatment of idiopathic sudden sensorineural hearing loss. *Otology and Neurotology, 29*(4), 453–460.

Bauer, C. A. (2004). Mechanisms of tinnitus generation. *Current Opinions in Otolaryngology Head and Neck Surgery, 12*(5), 413–417.

Bauman, N. G. (2004). Musical ear syndrome. *Hearing Health, 20*(4), 1–3.

Beck, J. S. (1995). *Cognitive therapy: Basics and beyond.* New York, NY: Guilford.

Berry, J. A., Gold, S. L., Frederick, E. A., Gray, W. C., & Staecker, H. (2002). Patient-based outcomes in patients with primary tinnitus undergoing tinnitus retraining therapy. *Archives of Otolaryngology, Head and Neck Surgery, 128*(10), 1153–1157.

Blyth, F. M., March, L. M., Nicholas, M. K., & Cousins, M. J. (2005). Self-management of chronic pain: A population-based study. *Pain, 113*(3), 285–292.

Brown, G. K., Henriques, G. R., Sosdjan, D., & Beck, A. T. (2004). Suicide intent and accurate expectations of lethality: Predictors of medical lethality of suicide attempts. *Journal of Consulting Clinical Psychology, 72*(6), 1170–1174.

Brown, S. C. (1990). *Older Americans and tinnitus: A demographic study and chartbook. GRI Monograph Series A, No. 2.* Washington, DC: Gallaudet Research Institute, Gallaudet University.

Brozoski, T. J., Bauer, C. A., & Caspary, D. M. (2002). Elevated fusiform cell activity in the dorsal cochlear nucleus of chinchillas with psychophysical evidence of tinnitus. *Journal of Neuroscience, 22*(6), 2383–2390.

Cacace, A. T. (2003). Expanding the biological basis of tinnitus: Crossmodal origins and the role of neuroplasticity. *Hearing Research, 175*(1–2), 112–132.

Choong, C., Hunter, M. D., & Woodruff, P. W. (2007). Auditory hallucinations in those populations that do not suffer from schizophrenia. *Current Psychiatry Reports, 9*(3), 206–212.

Coles, R. R. A. (1984). Epidemiology of tinnitus: (2) demographic and clinical features. *Journal of Laryngology and Otology, Supplementum 9*, 195–202.

Coles, R. R. A. (1995). Classification of causes, mechanisms of patient disturbance, and associated counseling. In J. A. Vernon & A. R. Moller (Eds.), *Mechanisms of tinnitus* (pp. 11–19). Boston, MA: Allyn & Bacon.

Coles, R. R. A. (1996). Tinnitus: Epidemiology, aetiology and classification. In G. Reich & J. A. Vernon (Eds.), *Proceedings of the Fifth International Tinnitus Seminar 1995* (pp. 25–29). Portland, OR: American Tinnitus Association.

Coles, R. R. A. (2000). Medicolegal issues. In R. S. Tyler (Ed.), *Tinnitus handbook* (pp. 399–417). San Diego, CA: Singular Publishing Group.

Dauman, R., & Tyler, R. S. (1992). Some considerations on the classification of tinnitus. In J.-M. Aran & R. Dauman (Eds.), *Proceedings of the Fourth International Tinnitus Seminar, Bordeaux, France* (pp. 225–229). Amsterdam/New York, NY: Kugler.

Davis, A., & Refaie, A. E. (2000). Epidemiology of tinnitus. In R. Tyler (Ed.), *Tinnitus handbook* (pp. 1–23). San Diego, CA: Singular Publishing Group.

Davis, A. C. (1995). *Hearing in adults.* London, England: Whurr.

Davis, P. B. (2006). Music and the acoustic desensitization protocol for tinnitus. In R. S. Tyler (Ed.), *Tinnitus treatment: Clinical protocols* (pp. 146–160). New York, NY: Thieme Medical.

Davis, P. B., Paki, B., & Hanley, P. J. (2007). Neuromonics tinnitus treatment: Third clinical trial. *Ear and Hearing, 28*(2), 242–259.

Del Bo, L., & Ambrosetti, U. (2007). Hearing aids for the treatment of tinnitus. *Progress in Brain Research, 166*, 341–345.

DiSorga, R. M. (2001). Adverse drug reactions and audiology practice. *Audiology Today, 13*(Special Issue: Drug Reactions), 2–7.

Doak, C. C., Doak, L. G., & Root, J. H. (1996). *Teaching patients with low literacy skills*. Philadelphia, PA: J.B. Lippincott.

Dobie, R. A. (2003). Depression and tinnitus. *Otolaryngologic Clinics of North America, 36*(2), 383–388.

Dobie, R. A. (2004a). Clinical trials and drug therapy for tinnitus. In J. B. Snow (Ed.), *Tinnitus: Theory and management* (pp. 266–277). Lewiston, NY: BC Decker.

Dobie, R. A. (2004b). Overview: Suffering from tinnitus. In J. B. Snow (Ed.), *Tinnitus: Theory and management* (pp. 1–7). Lewiston, NY: BC Decker.

Douek, E., & Reid, J. (1968). The diagnostic value of tinnitus pitch. *Journal of Laryngology and Otology, 82*, 1039–1042.

du Feu, M., & McKenna, P. J. (1999). Prelingually profoundly deaf schizophrenic patients who hear voices: A phenomenological analysis. *Acta Psychiatrica Scandinavica, 99*(6), 453–459.

Eggermont, J. J. (1990). On the pathophysiology of tinnitus; a review and a peripheral model. *Hearing Research, 48*, 111–124.

Eggermont, J. J. (2000). Physiological mechanisms and neural models. In R. Tyler (Ed.), *Tinnitus handbook* (pp. 85–122). San Diego, CA: Singular Publishing Group.

Eggermont, J. J. (2004). The auditory cortex and tinnitus. In J. B. Snow (Ed.), *Tinnitus: Theory and management* (pp. 171–188). Lewiston, NY: BC Decker.

Eggermont, J. J., & Roberts, L. E. (2004). The neuroscience of tinnitus. *Trends in Neuroscience, 27*(11), 676–682.

Erlandsson, S. (2000). Psychological profiles of tinnitus patients. In R. S. Tyler (Ed.), *Tinnitus handbook* (pp. 25–57). San Diego, CA: Singular Publishing Group.

Erlandsson, S. I., Hallberg, L. R. M., & Axelsson, A. (1992). Psychological and audiological correlates of perceived tinnitus severity. *Audiology, 31*, 168–179.

Fausti, S. A., Henry, J. A., & Frey, R. H. (1995). Ototoxicity. In J. L. Northern (Ed.), *Hearing disorders* (pp. 149–164). Boston, MA: Allyn & Bacon.

Fisch, U. (1970). Transtemporal surgery of the internal auditory canal: Report of 92 cases, technique, indications and results. *Advances in Oto-Rhino-Laryngology, 17*, 203–240.

Folmer, R. L., & Carroll, J. R. (2006). Long-term effectiveness of ear-level devices for tinnitus. *Otolaryngology, Head and Neck Surgery, 134*(1), 132–137.

Folmer, R. L., & Griest, S. E. (2000). Tinnitus and insomnia. *American Journal of Otolaryngology, 21*(5), 287–293.

Formby, C., & Gold, S. L. (2002). Modification of loudness discomfort level: Evidence for adaptive chronic auditory gain and its clinical relevance. *Seminars in Hearing, 23*, 21–35.

Formby, C., Sherlock, L. P., & Gold, S. L. (2002). Adaptive recalibration of chronic auditory gain: interim findings. In R. Patuzzi (Ed.), *VIIth International Tinnitus Seminar Proceedings* (pp. 165–169). Perth, Australia: Physiology Dept., Univ. of Western Australia.

Fulton, R. T., & Lloyd, L. L. (1975). *Auditory assessment of the difficult-to-test*. Baltimore, MD: Williams & Williams.

Gazmararian, J. A., Baker, D. W., Williams, M. V., Parker, R. M., Scott, T. L., Green, D. C., . . . Koplan, J. P. (1999). Health literacy among Medicare enrollees in a managed care organization. *Journal of the American Medical Association, 281*(6), 545–551.

Gold, S. L., Frederick, E. A., & Formby, C. (1999). Shifts in dynamic range for hyperacusis patients receiving tinnitus retraining therapy (TRT). In J. Hazell (Ed.), *Proceedings of the Sixth International Tinnitus Seminar 1999* (pp. 297–301). London, England: The Tinnitus and Hyperacusis Centre.

Goodhill, V., & Harris, I. (1979). Sudden hearing loss syndrome. In V. Goodhill (Ed.), *Ear diseases, deafness and dizziness*. New York, NY: Harper and Row.

Green, D. S. (1972). Pure tone air conduction thresholds. In J. Katz (Ed.), *Handbook of clinical audiology* (1st ed., pp. 67–86). Baltimore, MD: Williams & Wilkins.

Halford, J. B. S., & Anderson, S. D. (1991). Anxiety and depression in tinnitus sufferers. *Journal of Psychosometric Research, 35*, 383–390.

Hallam, R., Rachman, S., & Hinchcliffe, R. (1984). Psychological aspects of tinnitus. In S. Rachman (Ed.), *Contributions to medical psychology* (Vol. 3, pp. 31–53). Oxford, NY: Pergamon Press.

Hamid, M., & Trune, D. (2008). Issues, indications, and controversies regarding intratympanic steroid perfusion. *Current Opinion in Otolaryngology and Head Neck Surgery, 16*(5), 434–440.

Handscomb, L. (2006). Analysis of responses to individual items on the tinnitus handicap inventory according to severity of tinnitus handicap. *American Journal of Audiology, 15*(2), 102–107.

Harrop-Griffiths, J., Katon, W., Dobie, R., Sakai, C., & Russo, J. (1987). Chronic tinnitus: association with psychiatric diagnoses. *Journal of Psychosomatic Research, 31*(5), 613–621.

Hawton, K. (2001). Studying survivors of nearly lethal suicide attempts: An important strategy in suicide research. *Suicide and Life-Threatening Behavior, 32*(Suppl. 1), 76–84.

Hazell, J. (1998a). Incidence, classification, and models of tinnitus. In H. Ludman & T. Wright (Eds.), *Diseases of the ear* (pp. 185–195). London, England: Arnold.

Hazell, J. (1998b). Management of tinnitus. In H. Ludman & T. Wright (Eds.), *Diseases of the ear* (pp. 202–215). London, England: Arnold.

Hazell, J. (2003, 5 Jan). Things that go bump in the night. *International Tinnitus and Hyperacusis Society Newsletter*.

Hazell, J. W., Wood, S. M., Cooper, H. R., Stephens, S. D., Corcoran, A. L., Coles, R. R., . . . Sheldrake, J. B. (1985). A clinical study of tinnitus maskers. *British Journal of Audiology, 19*, 65–146.

Hazell, J. W. P. (1990). Tinnitus II: Surgical management of conditions associated with tinnitus and somatosounds. *Journal of Otolaryngology, 19*, 6–10.

Hazell, J. W. P. (1995). Models of tinnitus: Generation, perception, clinical implications. In J. A. Vernon & A. R. Møller (Eds.), *Mechanisms of tinnitus* (pp. 57–72). Boston, MA: Allyn & Bacon.

Hazell, J. W. P. (1999). The TRT method in practice. In J. Hazell (Ed.), *Proceedings of the Sixth International Tinnitus Seminar 1999* (pp. 92–98). London, England: The Tinnitus and Hyperacusis Centre.

Heller, A. J. (2003). Classification and epidemiology of tinnitus. *Otolaryngologic Clinics of North America, 36*(2), 239–248.

Henry, J. A. (2004). Audiologic assessment. In J. B. Snow (Ed.), *Tinnitus: Theory and management* (pp. 220–236). Lewiston, NY: BC Decker.

Henry, J. A., Dennis, K., & Schechter, M. A. (2005). General review of tinnitus: Prevalence, mechanisms, effects, and management. *Journal of Speech, Language, and Hearing Research, 48*(5), 1204–1234.

Henry, J. A., Loovis, C., Montero, M., Kaelin, C., Anselmi, K. A., Coombs, R., . . . James, K. E. (2007). Randomized clinical trial: Group counseling based on tinnitus retraining therapy. *Journal of Rehabilitation Research and Development, 44*(1), 21–32.

Henry, J. A., & Meikle, M. B. (1999). Pulsed versus continuous tones for evaluating the loudness of tinnitus. *Journal of the American Academy of Audiology, 10*, 261–272.

Henry, J. A., Rheinsburg, B., & Zaugg, T. (2004). Comparison of custom sounds for achieving tinnitus relief. *Journal of the American Academy of Audiology, 15*, 585–598.

Henry, J. A., Schechter, M. A., Nagler, S. M., & Fausti, S. A. (2002). Comparison of tinnitus masking and tinnitus retraining therapy. *Journal of the American Academy of Audiology, 13*, 559–581.

Henry, J. A., Schechter, M. A., Zaugg, T. L., Griest, S. E., Jastreboff, P. J., Vernon, J. A., . . . Stewart, B. J. (2006a). Clinical trial to compare tinnitus masking and tinnitus retraining therapy. *Acta Otolaryngology Supplementum, 126*, 64–69.

Henry, J. A., Schechter, M. A., Zaugg, T. L., Griest, S. E., Jastreboff, P. J., Vernon, J. A., . . . Stewart, B. J. (2006b). Outcomes of clinical trial: Tinnitus masking versus tinnitus retraining therapy. *Journal of the American Academy of Audiology, 17*, 104–132.

Henry, J. A., Trune, D. R., Robb, M. J. A., & Jastreboff, P. J. (2007a). *Tinnitus retraining therapy: Clinical guidelines*. San Diego, CA: Plural Publishing.

Henry, J. A., Trune, D. R., Robb, M. J. A., & Jastreboff, P. J. (2007b). *Tinnitus retraining therapy: Patient counseling guide*. San Diego, CA: Plural Publishing.

Henry, J. A., Zaugg, T. L., Myers, P. J., & Kendall, C. J. (2009). *How to manage your tinnitus: A step-by-step workbook* (2 ed.). Portland, OR: VA National Center for Rehabilitative Auditory Research.

Henry, J. A., Zaugg, T. L., Myers, P. J., Kendall, C. J., & Turbin, M. B. (2009). Principles and application of counseling used in progressive audiologic tinnitus management. *Noise and Health, 11*(42), 33–48.

Henry, J. A., Zaugg, T. L., Myers, P. J., & Schechter, M. A. (2008a). Progressive audiologic tinnitus management. *Asha Leader, 13*(8), 14–17.

Henry, J. A., Zaugg, T. L., Myers, P. J., & Schechter, M. A. (2008b). The role of audiologic evaluation in progressive audiologic tinnitus management. *Trends in Amplification, 12*(3), 169–184.

Henry, J. A., Zaugg, T. L., Myers, P. J., & Schechter, M. A. (2008c). Using therapeutic sound with progressive audiologic tinnitus management. *Trends in Amplification, 12*(3), 185–206.

Henry, J. A., Zaugg, T. L., Myers, P. M., & Kendall, C. J. (2010a). *How to manage your tinnitus: A step-by-step workbook* (3 ed.). San Diego, CA: Plural Publishing.

Henry, J. A., Zaugg, T. L., Myers, P. M., & Kendall, C. J. (2010b). *Progressive tinnitus management: Counseling guide*. San Diego, CA: Plural Publishing.

Henry, J. A., Zaugg, T. L., & Schechter, M. A. (2005a). Clinical guide for audiologic tinnitus management I: Assessment. *American Journal of Audiology, 14*, 21–48.

Henry, J. A., Zaugg, T. L., & Schechter, M. A. (2005b). Clinical guide for audiologic tinnitus management II: Treatment. *American Journal of Audiology, 14*, 49–70.

Henry, J. L., & Wilson, P. H. (1996). The psychological management of tinnitus: Comparison of a combined cognitive educational program, education alone and a waiting-list control. *International Tinnitus Journal, 2*, 9–20.

Henry, J. L., & Wilson, P. H. (1998). Psychological treatments for tinnitus. In J. A. Vernon (Ed.), *Tinnitus treatment and relief* (pp. 99–115). Boston, MA: Allyn & Bacon.

Henry, J. L., & Wilson, P. H. (2001). *The psychological management of chronic tinnitus*. Boston, MA: Allyn & Bacon.

Henry, J. L., & Wilson, P. H. (2002). *Tinnitus: A self-management guide for the ringing in your ears*. Boston, MA: Allyn & Bacon.

Herraiz, C., Hernandez, F. J., Plaza, G., & de los Santos, G. (2005). Long-term clinical trial of tinnitus retraining therapy. *Otolaryngology, Head and Neck Surgery, 133*(5), 774–779.

Herraiz, C., Hernandez, F. J., Toledano, A., & Aparicio, J. M. (2007). Tinnitus retraining therapy: Prognosis factors. *American Journal of Otolaryngology, 28*(4), 225–229.

Hochberg, I., & Waltzman, S. (1972). Comparison of pulsed and continuous tone thresholds in patients with tinnitus. *Audiology, 11*, 337–342.

Hoffman, B. M., Papas, R. K., Chatkoff, D. K., & Kerns, R. D. (2007). Meta-analysis of psychological interventions for chronic low back pain. *Health Psychology, 26*(1), 1–9.

Hoffman, H. J., & Reed, G. W. (2004). Epidemiology of tinnitus. In J. B. Snow (Ed.), *Tinnitus: Theory and management* (pp. 16–41). Lewiston, NY: BC Decker.

Hofmann, S. G., & Smits, J. A. (2008). Cognitive-behavioral therapy for adult anxiety disorders: a meta-analysis of randomized placebo-controlled trials. *Journal of Clinical Psychiatry, 69*(4), 621–632.

House, J. W., & Brackmann, D. E. (1981). Tinnitus: Surgical management. In Evered & Lawrenson (Eds.), *Tinnitus (Ciba Foundation Symposium 85)* (pp. 204–216). London, England: Pitman.

Howard, D. H., Gazmararian, J., & Parker, R. M. (2005). The impact of low health literacy on the medical costs of Medicare managed care enrollees. *American Journal of Medicine, 118*(4), 371–377.

Hugdahl, K., Loberg, E. M., Jorgensen, H. A., Lundervold, A., Lund, A., Green, M. F., & Rund, B. (2008). Left hemisphere lateralisation of auditory hallucinations in schizophrenia: A dichotic listening study. *Cognition Neuropsychiatry, 13*(2), 166–179.

Humes, L. E., Joellenbeck, L. M., & Durch, J. S. (Eds.). (2006). *Noise and military service: Implications for hear-*

ing loss and tinnitus. Washington, DC: The National Academies Press.

Jakes, S. C., Hallam, R. S., Chambers, C., & Hinchcliffe, R. (1985). A factor analytical study of tinnitus complaint behaviour. *Audiology, 24*, 195–206.

Jastreboff, M. M., & Jastreboff, P. J. (2002). Decreased sound tolerance and Tinnitus retraining therapy (TRT). *Australian and New Zealand Journal of Audiology, 24*, 74–81.

Jastreboff, P. J. (1990). Phantom auditory perception (tinnitus): Mechanisms of generation and perception. *Neuroscience Research, 8*, 221–254.

Jastreboff, P. J. (1995). Tinnitus as a phantom perception: Theories and clinical implications. In J. A. Vernon & A. R. Moller (Eds.), *Mechanisms of tinnitus* (pp. 73–93). Boston, MA: Allyn & Bacon.

Jastreboff, P. J. (2000). Tinnitus habituation therapy (THT) and tinnitus retraining therapy (TRT). In R. S. Tyler (Ed.), *Tinnitus handbook* (pp. 357–376). San Diego, CA: Singular Publishing Group.

Jastreboff, P. J. (2004). The neurophysiological model of tinnitus. In J. B. Snow (Ed.), *Tinnitus: Theory and management* (pp. 96–107). Lewiston, NY: BC Decker.

Jastreboff, P. J., & Hazell, J. W. P. (1998). Treatment of tinnitus based on a neurophysiological model. In J. A. Vernon (Ed.), *Tinnitus treatment and relief* (pp. 201–217). Boston, MA: Allyn & Bacon.

Jastreboff, P. J., & Hazell, J. W. P. (2004). *Tinnitus retraining therapy: Implementing the neurophysiological model*. New York, NY: Cambridge University Press.

Jastreboff, P. J., & Jastreboff, M. M. (2000). Tinnitus retraining therapy (TRT) as a method for treatment of tinnitus and hyperacusis patients. *Journal of the American Academy of Audiology, 11*, 162–177.

Jastreboff, P. J., & Jastreboff, M. M. (2004). Decreased sound tolerance. In J. B. Snow (Ed.), *Tinnitus: Theory and management* (pp. 8–15). Lewiston, NY: BC Decker.

Jeyakumar, A., Francis, D., & Doerr, T. (2006). Treatment of idiopathic sudden sensorineural hearing loss. *Acta Otolaryngologica, 126*(7), 708–713.

Johns, M. W. (1991). A new method for measuring daytime sleepiness: The Epworth sleepiness scale. *Sleep, 14*(6), 540–545.

Johnson, M. H. (2005). How does distraction work in the management of pain? *Current Pain and Headaches Report, 9*(2), 90–95.

Johnson, R. M. (1998). The masking of tinnitus. In J. A. Vernon (Ed.), *Tinnitus treatment and relief* (pp. 164–186). Boston, MA: Allyn & Bacon.

Kaltenbach, J. A. (2000). Neurophysiologic mechanisms of tinnitus. *Journal of the American Academy of Audiology, 11*(3), 125–137.

Kaltenbach, J. A., & Afman, C. E. (2000). Hyperactivity in the dorsal cochlear nucleus after intense sound exposure and its resemblance to tone-evoked activity: A physiological model for tinnitus. *Hearing Research, 140*(1–2), 165–172.

Kaltenbach, J. A., Rachel, J. D., Mathog, T. A., Zhang, J., Falzarano, P. R., & Lewandowski, M. (2002). Cisplatin-induced hyperactivity in the dorsal cochlear nucleus and its relation to outer hair cell loss: Relevance to tinnitus. *Journal of Neurophysiology, 88*(2), 699–714.

Kaltenbach, J. A., Zhang, J., & Zacharek, M. A. (2004). Neural correlates of tinnitus. In J. B. Snow (Ed.), *Tinnitus: Theory and management* (pp. 141–161). Lewiston, NY: BC Decker.

Kessels, R. P. (2003). Patients' memory for medical information. *Journal of the Royal Society of Medicine, 96*(5), 219–222.

Kessler, R. C., Borges, G., & Walters, E. E. (1999). Prevalence of and risk factors for lifetime suicide attempts in the National Comorbidity Survey. *Archives of General Psychiatry, 56*(7), 617–626.

Kiang, N. Y. S., Moxon, E. C., & Levine, R. A. (1970). Auditory-nerve activity in cats with normal and abnormal cochleas. In G. E. W. Wolstenholme & J. Knight (Eds.), *Sensorineural hearing loss* (pp. 241–273). London, England: J. & A. Churchill.

Kirsch, C. A., Blanchard, E. B., & Parnes, S. M. (1989). Psychological characteristics of individuals high and low in their ability to cope with tinnitus. *Psychosomatic Medicine, 51*, 209–217.

Kraemer, D. J., Macrae, C. N., Green, A. E., & Kelley, W. M. (2005). Musical imagery: Sound of silence activates auditory cortex. *Nature, 434*(7030), 158.

Kroner-Herwig, B., Frenzel, A., Fritsche, G., Schilkowsky, G., & Esser, G. (2003). The management of chronic tinnitus: Comparison of an outpatient cognitive-behavioral group training to minimal-contact interventions. *Journal of Psychosomatic Research, 54*(4), 381–389.

Levine, R. A. (2004). Somatic tinnitus. In J. B. Snow (Ed.), *Tinnitus: Theory and management* (pp. 108–124). Lewiston, NY: BC Decker.

Lichtenstein, M. J., Bess, F. H., Logan, S. A., & Burger, M. C. (1990). Deriving criteria for hearing impairment in the elderly: A functional approach. *Journal of the American Academy of Audiology, 1*(1), 11–22.

Lockwood, A. H., Burkard, R. F., & Salvi, R. J. (2004). Imaging tinnitus. In J. B. Snow (Ed.), *Tinnitus: The-*

ory and management (pp. 253–264). Lewiston, NY: BC Decker.

Margolis, R. H. (2004). Audiology information counseling—What do patients remember? *Audiology Today, 16*(2), 14–15.

Martinez Devesa, P., Waddell, A., Perera, R., & Theodoulou, M. (Eds.). (2007). *Cognitive behavioural therapy for tinnitus (Review), Cochrane Database of Systematic Reviews 2007, Issue 1.*

Mayeaux, E. J., Jr., Murphy, P. W., Arnold, C., Davis, T. C., Jackson, R. H., & Sentell, T. (1996). Improving patient education for patients with low literacy skills. *American Family Physician, 53*(1), 205–211.

Meikle, M., & Walsh, E. T. (1984). Characteristics of tinnitus and related observations in over 1800 tinnitus patients. In *Proceedings of the Second International Tinnitus Seminar, New York 1983. The Journal of Laryngology and Otology, Suppl. 9* (pp. 17–21). Ashford, Kent: Invicta Press.

Meikle, M. B. (1995). The interaction of central and peripheral mechanisms in tinnitus. In J. A. Vernon & A. R. Møller (Eds.), *Mechanisms of tinnitus* (pp. 181–206). Boston, MA: Allyn & Bacon.

Meikle, M. B., Creedon, T. A., & Griest, S. E. (2004). *Tinnitus archive, 2nd ed.* Retrieved February 15, 2010, from http://www.tinnitusarchive.org/

Meikle, M. B., Vernon, J., & Johnson, R. M. (1984). The perceived severity of tinnitus. *Otolaryngology-Head and Neck Surgery, 92*(6), 689–696.

Mensing, C. R., & Norris, S. L. (2003). Group education in diabetes: Effectiveness and implementation. *Diabetes Spectrum, 16*(2), 96–103.

Merchant, S. N., Adams, J. C., & Nadol, J. B., Jr. (2005). Pathology and pathophysiology of idiopathic sudden sensorineural hearing loss. *Otology and Neurotology, 26*(2), 151–160.

Mineau, S. M., & Schlauch, R. S. (1997). Threshold measurement for patients with tinnitus: Pulsed or continuous tones. *American Journal of Audiology, 6*, 52–56.

Moffat, D. A., & Hardy, D. G. (1989). Surgical management of large glomus jugulare tumours: Infra- and trans-temporal approach. *Journal of Laryngology and Otology, 103*(12), 1167–1180.

Møller, A. R. (1984). Pathophysiology of tinnitus. *Annals of Otology, Rhinology, and Laryngology, 93*, 39–44.

Møller, A. R. (1987). Similarities between chronic pain and tinnitus. *American Journal of Otology, 18*, 577–585.

Møller, A. R. (1995). Pathophysiology of tinnitus. In J. A. Vernon & A. R. Møller (Eds.), *Mechanisms of tinnitus* (pp. 207–217). Needham Heights, MA: Allyn & Bacon.

Møller, A. R. (2000). Similarities between severe tinnitus and chronic pain. *Journal of the American Academy of Audiology, 11*, 115–124.

Møller, A. R. (2003). Pathophysiology of tinnitus. *Otolaryngologic Clinics of North America, 36*(2), 249–266, v–vi.

Newman, C. W., Jacobson, G. P., & Spitzer, J. B. (1996). Development of the tinnitus handicap inventory. *Archives of Otolaryngology-Head and Neck Surgery, 122*, 143–148.

Newman, C. W., & Sandridge, S. A. (2004). Tinnitus questionnaires. In J. B. Snow (Ed.), *Tinnitus: Theory and management* (pp. 237–254). Lewiston, NY: BC Decker.

Newman, C. W., & Sandridge, S. A. (2005). Incorporating group and individual sessions into a tinnitus management clinic. In R. S. Tyler (Ed.), *Tinnitus treatment: Clinical protocols* (pp. 187–197). New York, NY: Thieme.

Newman, C. W., Sandridge, S. A., & Bolek, L. (2008). Development and psychometric adequacy of the screening version of the tinnitus handicap inventory. *Otology and Neurotology, 29*(3), 276–281.

Newman, C. W., Sandridge, S. A., & Jacobson, G. P. (1998). Psychometric adequacy of the Tinnitus Handicap Inventory (THI) for evaluating treatment outcome. *Journal of the American Academy of Audiology, 9*, 153–160.

Newman, C. W., Weinstein, B. E., Jacobson, G. P., & Hug, G. A. (1990). The hearing handicap inventory for adults: Psychometric adequacy and audiometric correlates. *Ear and Hearing, 11*, 430–433.

Newman, S., Mulligan, K., & Steed, L. (2001). What is meant by self-management and how can its efficacy be established? *Rheumatology (Oxford), 40*(1), 1–4.

Nicolson, S. E., Mayberg, H. S., Pennell, P. B., & Nemeroff, C. B. (2006). Persistent auditory hallucinations that are unresponsive to antipsychotic drugs. *American Journal of Psychiatry, 163*(7), 1153–1159.

Nielsen-Bohlman, L., Panzer, A. M., & Kindig, D. A. (Eds.). (2004). *Health literacy: A prescription to end confusion*. Washington, DC: Institute of Medicine of the National Academies.

Nuttall, A. L., Meikle, M. B., & Trune, D. R. (2004). Peripheral processes involved in tinnitus. In J. B. Snow (Ed.), *Tinnitus: Theory and management* (pp. 52–68). Lewiston, NY: BC Decker.

Patuzzi, R. (2002). Outer hair cells, EP regulation and tinnitus. In R. Patuzzi (Ed.), *Seventh Interna-*

tional Tinnitus Seminar Proceedings. Perth, Australia: Physiology Department, University of Western Australia.

Penner, M. J., & Bilger, R. C. (1995). Psychophysical observations and the origin of tinnitus. In J. A. Vernon & A. R. Moller (Eds.), *Mechanisms of tinnitus* (pp. 219–230). Needham Heights, MA: Allyn & Bacon.

Perry, B. P., & Gantz, B. J. (2000). Medical and surgical evaluation and management of tinnitus. In R. S. Tyler (Ed.), *Tinnitus handbook* (pp. 221–241). San Diego, CA: Singular Publishing Group.

Prins, A., Ouimette, P., Kimerling, R., Cameron, R. P., Hugelshofer, D. S., Shaw-Hegwer, J., . . . Sheikh, J. I. (2004). The primary care PTSD screen (PC-PTSD): Development and operating characteristics. *Primary Care Psychiatry, 9*, 9–14.

Puel, J. L., & Guitton, M. J. (2007). Salicylate-induced tinnitus: Molecular mechanisms and modulation by anxiety. *Progressive Brain Research, 166*, 141–146.

Pulec, J. L. (1984). Tinnitus: Surgical therapy. *American Journal of Otology, 5*, 479–480.

Rachel, J. D., Kaltenbach, J. A., & Janisse, J. (2002). Increases in spontaneous neural activity in the hamster dorsal cochlear nucleus following cisplatin treatment: A possible basis for cisplatin-induced tinnitus. *Hearing Research, 164*(1–2), 206–214.

Robinson, S. K., Viirre, E. S., & Stein, M. B. (2004). Antidepressant therapy for tinnitus. In J. B. Snow (Ed.), *Tinnitus: Theory and management* (pp. 278–293). Lewiston, NY: BC Decker.

Rollnick, S., Mason, P., & Butler, C. (1999). *Health behavior change: A guide for practitioners*. Philadelphia, PA: Elsevier.

Sacks, O. (2008). *Musicophilia: Tales of music and the brain*. New York, NY: Random House.

Salvi, R. J., Lockwood, A. H., & Burkard, R. (2000). Neural plasticity and tinnitus. In R. Tyler (Ed.), *Tinnitus handbook* (pp. 123–148). San Diego, CA: Singular Publishing Group.

Saltzman, M., & Ersner, M. S. (1947). A hearing aid for relief of tinnitus aurium. *Laryngoscope, 57*, 358–366.

Sandridge, S. A., & Newman, C. W. (2005). Benefits of group informational counseling. In R. Dauman (Ed.), *VIIIth International Tinnitus Seminar* (p. 106). Bordeaux, France: ENT Dept., University Hospital of Bordeaux.

Schechter, M. A., & Henry, J. A. (2002). Assessment and treatment of tinnitus patients using a "masking approach." *Journal of the American Academy of Audiology, 13*, 545–558.

Schleuning, A. J., Johnson, R. M., & Vernon, J. A. (1980). Evaluation of a tinnitus masking program: a follow-up study of 598 patients. *Ear and Hearing, 1*, 71–74.

Schonauer, K., Achtergarde, D., Gotthardt, U., & Folkerts, H. W. (1998). Hallucinatory modalities in prelingually deaf schizophrenic patients: A retrospective analysis of 67 cases. *Acta Psychiatrica Scandinavica, 98*(5), 377–383.

Schuknecht, H. F. (1993). *Pathology of the ear*. Boston, MA: Lea & Febiger.

Schwaber, M. K. (2003). Medical evaluation of tinnitus. *Otolaryngologic Clinics of North America, 36*(2), 287–292, vi.

Scott, B., Lindberg, P., Melin, L., & Lyttkens, L. (1990). Predictors of tinnitus discomfort, adaptation and subjective loudness. *British Journal of Audiology, 24*, 51–62.

Seal, M. L., Aleman, A., & McGuire, P. K. (2004). Compelling imagery, unanticipated speech and deceptive memory: Neurocognitive models of auditory verbal hallucinations in schizophrenia. *Cognitive Neuropsychiatry, 9*(1–2), 43–72.

Searchfield, G. D. (2005). Hearing aids and tinnitus. In R. S. Tyler (Ed.), *Tinnitus treatment: Clinical protocols* (pp. 161–175). New York, NY: Thieme.

Shapiro, D. E., Boggs, S. R., Melamed, B. G., & Graham-Pole, J. (1992). The effect of varied physician affect on recall, anxiety, and perceptions in women at risk for breast cancer: An analogue study. *Health Psychology, 11*(1), 61–66.

Sindhusake, D., Golding, M., Newall, P., Rubin, G., Jakobsen, K., & Mitchell, P. (2003). Risk factors for tinnitus in a population of older adults: The blue mountains hearing study. *Ear and Hearing, 24*(6), 501–507.

Sindhusake, D., Mitchell, P., Newall, P., Golding, M., Rochtchina, E., & Rubin, G. (2003). Prevalence and characteristics of tinnitus in older adults: The Blue Mountains Hearing Study. *International Journal of Audiology, 42*(5), 289–294.

Sismanis, A. (1998). Pulsatile tinnitus. In J. A. Vernon (Ed.), *Tinnitus treatment and relief* (pp. 28–33). Boston, MA: Allyn & Bacon.

Sismanis, A. (2003). Pulsatile tinnitus. *Otolaryngologic Clinics of North America, 36*(2), 389–402, viii.

Sismanis, A. (2007). Evaluation and management of pulsatile tinnitus. In G. B. Hughes & M. L. Pensak (Eds.), *Clinical Otology*. New York, NY: Thieme.

Sommer, I. E., Daalman, K., Rietkerk, T., Diederen, K. M., Bakker, S., Wijkstra, J., & Boks, M. P. (2008). Healthy individuals with auditory verbal hallucinations; who are they? Psychiatric assessments of a selected sample of 103 subjects. *Schizophrenia Bulletin*.

Stephens, S., & Corcoran, A. (1985). A controlled study of tinnitus masking. *British Journal of Audiology, 19*, 159–167.

Stetler, C. B., Legro, M. W., Wallace, C. M., Bowman, C., Guihan, M., Hagedorn, H., . . . Smith, J. L. (2006). The role of formative evaluation in implementation research and the QUERI experience. *Journal of General Internal Medicine, 21*(Suppl. 2), S1–S8.

Stewart, M., Brown, J. B., Donner, A., McWhinney, I. R., Oates, J., Weston, W. W., Jordan, J. (2000). The impact of patient-centered care on outcomes. *Journal of Family Practice, 49*, 796–804.

Surr, R. K., Kolb, J. A., Cord, M. T., & Garrus, N. P. (1999). Tinnitus handicap inventory (THI) as a hearing aid outcome measure. *Journal of the American Academy of Audiology, 10*(9), 489–495.

Surr, R. K., Montgomery, A. A., & Mueller, H. G. (1985). Effect of amplification on tinnitus among new hearing aid users. *Ear and Hearing, 6*(2), 71–75.

Sweetow, R. W. (1996). Tinnitus. In J. L. Northern (Ed.), *Hearing disorders* (pp. 299–308). Boston, MA: Allyn & Bacon.

Sweetow, R. W. (2000). Cognitive-behavior modification. In R. S. Tyler (Ed.), *Tinnitus handbook* (pp. 297–311). San Diego, CA: Singular Publishing Group.

Trotter, M. I., & Donaldson, I. (2008). Hearing aids and tinnitus therapy: A 25-year experience. *Journal of Laryngology and Otology*, 1–5.

Trune, D. R. (2004). Ion homeostasis and inner ear disease. In M. Hamid & A. Sismanis (Eds.), *Medical otology and neurotology*. New York, NY: Thieme.

Tyler, R. S. (2006). Neurophysiological models, psychological models, and treatments for tinnitus. In R. S. Tyler (Ed.), *Tinnitus treatment: Clinical protocols* (pp. 1–22). San Diego, CA: Thieme.

Tyler, R. S., & Baker, L. J. (1983). Difficulties experienced by tinnitus sufferers. *Journal of Speech and Hearing Disorders, 48*, 150–154.

Ventry, I. M., & Weinstein, B. E. (1982). The Hearing Handicap Inventory for the Elderly: A new tool. *Ear and Hearing, 3*, 128–134.

Ventry, I. M., & Weinstein, B. E. (1983). Identification of elderly people with hearing problems. *Asha, 25*(7), 37–42.

Vernon, J. (1976). The use of masking for relief of tinnitus. In H. Silverstein & H. Norrell (Eds.), *Neurological Surgery of the Ear: Volume II* (pp. 104–118). Birmingham, AL: Aesculapius Publishing.

Vernon, J. (1977). Attempts to relieve tinnitus. *Journal of the American Audiology Society, 2*, 124–131.

Vernon, J., & Schleuning, A. (1978). Tinnitus: A new management. *Laryngoscope, 88*, 413–419.

Vernon, J. A. (1976). The loudness (?) of tinnitus. *Hearing and Speech Action, 44*, 17–19.

Vernon, J. A. (1996). Is the claimed tinnitus real and is the claimed cause correct? In G. E. Reich & J. A. Vernon (Eds.), *Proceedings of the Fifth International Tinnitus Seminar, 1995* (pp. 395–396). Portland, OR: American Tinnitus Association.

Vernon, J. A. (1998). *Tinnitus treatment and relief*. Boston, MA: Allyn & Bacon.

Vernon, J. A. (2002). Hyperacusis: Testing, treatments and a possible mechanism. *Australian and New Zealand Journal of Audiology, 24*, 68–73.

Vernon, J. A., & Møller, A. R. (1995). *Mechanisms of tinnitus*. Boston, MA: Allyn & Bacon.

Vernon, J. A., & Press, L. (1998). Treatment for hyperacusis. In J. A. Vernon (Ed.), *Tinnitus treatment and relief* (pp. 223–227). Boston, MA: Allyn & Bacon.

Wackym, P. A., & Friedland, D. R. (2004). Otologic evaluation. In J. B. Snow (Ed.), *Tinnitus: Theory and management* (pp. 205–219). Lewiston, NY: B.C. Decker.

Weiss, B. D., Hart, G., McGee, D. L., & D'Estelle, S. (1992). Health status of illiterate adults: Relation between literacy and health status among persons with low literacy skills. *Journal of the American Board of Family Practice, 5*(3), 257–264.

Weiss, B. D., & Palmer, R. (2004). Relationship between health care costs and very low literacy skills in a medically needy and indigent Medicaid population. *Journal of the American Board of Family Practice, 17*(1), 44–47.

Wengel, S. P., Burke, W. J., & Holemon, D. (1989). Musical hallucinations. The sounds of silence? *Journal of the American Geriatric Society, 37*(2), 163–166.

Wilkinson, M. J., & Barczak, P. (1988). Psychiatric screening in general practice: Comparison of the general health questionnaire and the hospital anxiety depression scale. *Journal of the Royal College of General Practitioners, 38*(312), 311–313.

Williams, M. V., Davis, T., Parker, R. M., & Weiss, B. D. (2002). The role of health literacy in patient-physician communication. *Family Medicine, 34*(5), 383–389.

Williams, M. V., Parker, R. M., Baker, D. W., Parikh, N. S., Pitkin, K., Coates, W. C., & Nurss, J. R. (1995). Inadequate functional health literacy among patients at two public hospitals. *Journal of the American Medical Association, 274*(21), 1677–1682.

Wilson, P. H., Henry, J. L., & Nicholas, M. (1993). Cognitive methods in the management of chronic pain and tinnitus. *Australian Psychologist, 28*, 172–180.

Wilson, S. R. (1997). Individual versus group education: Is one better? *Patient Education and Counseling, 32*(Suppl. 1), S67–75.

Yantis, P. A. (1994). Puretone air-conduction threshold testing. In J. Katz (Ed.), *Handbook of Clinical Audiology* (pp. 97–108). Baltimore, MD: Williams & Wilkins.

Zacharek, M. A., Kaltenbach, J. A., Mathog, T. A., & Zhang, J. (2002). Effects of cochlear ablation on noise induced hyperactivity in the hamster dorsal cochlear nucleus: implications for the origin of noise induced tinnitus. *Hearing Research, 172*(1–2), 137–143.

Zaugg, T. L., Schechter, M. A., Fausti, S. A., & Henry, J. A. (2002). Difficulties caused by patients' misconceptions that hearing problems are due to tinnitus. In R. Patuzzi (Ed.), *Proceedings of the Seventh International Tinnitus Seminar* (pp. 226–228). Crawley, Australia: University of Western Australia.

Zigmond, A. S., & Snaith, R. P. (1983). The hospital anxiety and depression scale. *Acta Psychiatrica Scandinavica, 67*(6), 361–370.

APPENDIX

A

PTM

Progressive Tinnitus Management

PTM Flowchart

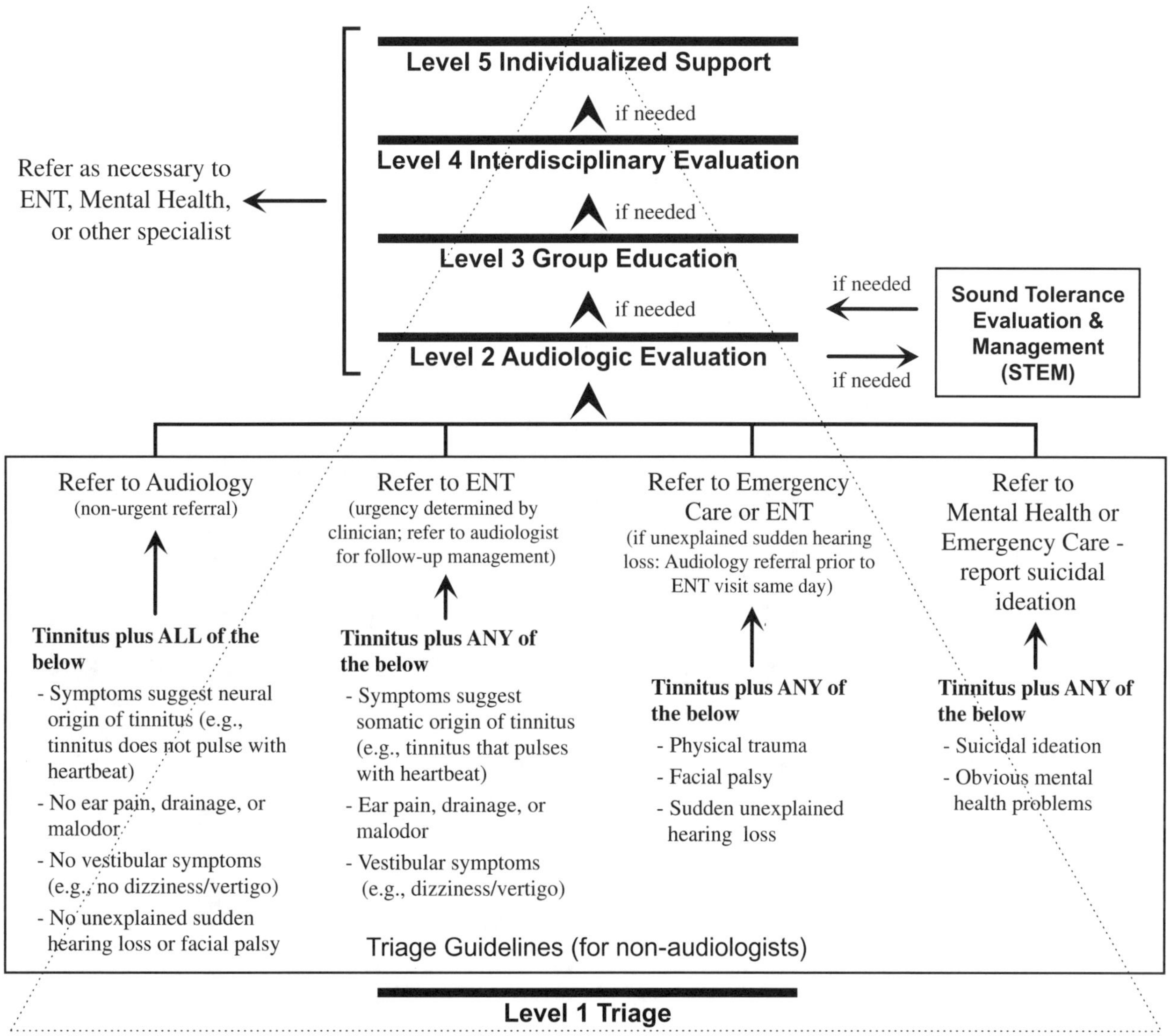

APPENDIX

B

PTM

Progressive Tinnitus Management

Tinnitus Triage Guidelines

(My Patient Complains About Tinnitus—What Should I Do?)

Tinnitus ("ringing in the ears") is experienced by 10 to 15% of the adult population. Of those, about one out of every five requires some degree of clinical intervention. When clinical intervention is required, often only some basic education is needed. However, some people with tinnitus have need for individualized care, or they have urgent medical issues. The following are general guidelines for triaging the patient who complains about tinnitus. Note that many symptoms that might be reported by patients are not included. For example, patients who report tinnitus may also report symptoms of head or neck injury/disease, or of TMJ disorder. These and other symptoms would indicate referral to appropriate specialists.

If the patient:	*Refer to:*
1. • Has physical trauma,facial palsy, or unexplained sudden hearing loss • Has any other urgent medical condition	Emergency Care or Otolaryngology (If unexplained sudden hearing loss—Audiology referral prior to Otolaryngology visit same day) *(emergency referral)*
2. • Has suicidal/homicidal ideations • Manifests obvious mental health problems	Emergency Care or Mental Health—report suicidal/homicidal ideation (*may be emergency*—if so, escort patient to Emergency Care or Mental Health)
3. Has ANY of the following: • Symptoms suggest somatic origin of tinnitus (example: tinnitus that pulses with heartbeat) • Ear pain, drainage, or malodor • Vestibular symptoms (example: dizziness/vertigo)	Otolaryngology (*urgency determined by clinician*; refer to audiologist for follow-up management)
4. Has ALL of the following: • Symptoms suggest neural origin of tinnitus (example: tinnitus that does not pulse with heartbeat) • No ear pain, drainage, or malodor • No vestibular symptoms (example:no dizziness/vertigo) • No unexplained sudden hearing loss or facial palsy	Audiology

APPENDIX

C

PTM

Progressive Tinnitus Management

Overview of Objectives and Procedures of the Level 2 Audiologic Evaluation

Determine need for:	*Assessment procedures:*	*Action needed:*
1. Referral for medical examination	Standard clinical procedures	Refer to otolaryngology
2. Hearing aids or assistive listening devices	Standard clinical procedures	Fit devices as appropriate
3. Level 3 Group Education	Discuss with patient the responses to the Tinnitus and Hearing Survey (primarily Section A) (Appendix D). If the patient is interested in attending a workshop that focuses on managing problems listed in section A then action is needed.	Schedule patient for group workshops (after fitting of any instruments)
4. Provision of Loudness Tolerance Handout: "What to Do When Everyday Sounds Are Too Loud" (Appendix E)	Review item 1 from Section C of the Tinnitus and Hearing Survey (Appendix D). If the patient reports at least a mild loudness tolerance problem, then action is needed.	Provide a copy of the handout to the patient with a brief explanation of its purpose
5. Assessment for a loudness tolerance problem	Discuss with the patient the responses to the Tinnitus and Hearing Survey (primarily item 2 from Section C) (Appendix D). If the patient reports that a loudness tolerance problem would make it difficult to attend a group education class, then action is needed.	Schedule the patient for a Sound Tolerance Evaluation and Management (STEM) appointment. Suspend Level 3 of PTM until the sound tolerance problem is resolved.
6. Mental health screening	Screening is done at Level 2 only if the patient exhibits behaviors or makes statements that would suggest the need for mental health screening	Refer patient to a mental health provider that is part of the "PTM or tinnitus team," or to primary care for mental health screening
7. Provision of self-help education workbook: *How to Manage Your Tinnitus: A Step-by-Step Workbook*	Patients who have problematic tinnitus should be advised to attend Level 3 Group Education. The workbook normally is provided to patients at the start of the first Level 3 workshop.	Issue a workbook at the end of Level 2 *only if the patient cannot or will not attend Level 3 Group Education.* If time permits, point out sections of the workbook that are applicable to the patient's situation.

PTM

Progressive Tinnitus Management

Tinnitus and Hearing Survey

A. Tinnitus	No, **not** a problem	Yes, a **small** problem	Yes, a **moderate** problem	Yes, a **big** problem	Yes, a **very big** problem	
Over the last week, tinnitus kept me from sleeping.	0	1	2	3	4	
Over the last week, tinnitus kept me from concentrating on reading.	0	1	2	3	4	
Over the last week, tinnitus kept me from relaxing.	0	1	2	3	4	
Over the last week, I couldn't get my mind off of my tinnitus.	0	1	2	3	4	Grand Total
Total of each column	___	___	___	___	___	☐

B. Hearing						
Over the last week, I couldn't understand what others were saying in noisy or crowded places.	0	1	2	3	4	
Over the last week, I couldn't understand what people were saying on TV or in movies.	0	1	2	3	4	
Over the last week, I couldn't understand people with soft voices.	0	1	2	3	4	
Over the last week, I couldn't understand what was being said in group conversations.	0	1	2	3	4	Grand Total
Total of each column	___	___	___	___	___	☐

C. Sound Tolerance					
Over the last week, everyday sounds were too loud for me.*	0	1	2	3	4
If you responded 1, 2, 3 or 4 to the statement above:					
Being in a meeting with 5 to 10 people would be too loud for me.*	0	1	2	3	4

*If sounds are too loud for you when wearing hearing aids, please tell your audiologist.

APPENDIX E

PTM

Progressive Tinnitus Management

What to Do When Everyday Sounds Are Too Loud

(Not related to using hearing aids)

Bill Smith is bothered by ***everyday sounds****. (This problem is sometimes called* ***hyperacusis****.) Kitchen sounds and the vacuum cleaner are too loud for him. He is bothered by road noise when he drives. It seems like everything at church is too loud. What should Bill do? Believe it or not, being around more sound can make things* ***better****! And, staying away from sound can make his problem* ***worse****! What??? He should add* ***more*** *sound??? Keep reading and we'll explain . . .*

There are three things you can do if everyday sounds are too loud for you.

1. Keep yourself surrounded with sound that is comfortable for you.
2. Listen to sounds that you enjoy as often as you can.
3. Only wear hearing protection when you really need to.

1. **Keep yourself surrounded with sound that is comfortable for you.**

Why should I keep myself surrounded with sound? Let's start by thinking about your eyes and how they adjust to light. Imagine sitting in a dark movie theater and then going outside into the daylight. Everything seems brighter to you than it does to people who were not sitting in the dark. Your eyes had adjusted to the dark and now they have to readjust to the daylight.

Your ears adjust to sound like your eyes adjust to light. If you stay away from sound, your ears will slowly adjust to the quiet. After a while, everyday sounds will seem louder and harder to tolerate. Avoiding sound will only make the problem worse.

If you keep yourself surrounded with sound, your ears will readjust. It will slowly become easier for you to tolerate everyday sounds. You should only use sounds that are comfortable for you. It usually takes at least a few weeks of being around sound for this change to happen.

How do I keep myself surrounded with sound? You can use any sound that is not annoying (the sound can be either neutral or pleasant). Here are some ideas:

- Listen to music at a comfortable level.
- Listen to radio shows.
- Play recordings of nature sounds.
- Keep a fan running.
- Use a tabletop water fountain.

Another choice: Some people wear small instruments in their ears that make a "shhh" sound. These instruments are called *in-the-ear noise generators* or *maskers*. Your audiologist can tell you more about them.

2. **Listen to sounds that you enjoy as often as you can.**

Why should I listen to sounds that I enjoy as often as I can? We just talked about the problem of everyday sounds being too loud (*hyperacusis*). Many people also have another problem: they just *don't like* certain sounds, but *not because they are too loud*. (This problem is sometimes called *misophonia*.) If you don't like certain sounds, you should make a point of listening to sounds that you enjoy. Spending time enjoying sound can help you get better at tolerating everyday sounds that you don't like.

3. **Only wear hearing protection when you really need to.**

Why should I use ear protection *only* when I really need to? When everyday sounds seem too loud, some people start using ear protection all the time. Remember that avoiding sound will make the problem worse. Only use ear protection when sounds are dangerously loud or uncomfortably loud. *As soon* as the sound around you is at a safe and comfortable level, take the ear protection off. The goal is to wear ear protection *only when needed*.

Use earplugs or earmuffs *only* when:

- sounds around you are uncomfortably loud
- you are around dangerously loud sounds like:
  - lawn mowers
  - loud concerts
  - power tools
  - guns
  - etc.

Is there any research?

Yes. In 2002 Formby, Sherlock, and Gold[1] studied *sound tolerance*.

- There were two groups of people:
  1. One group wore earplugs for 2 weeks.
  2. The other group wore in-the-ear sound generators ("maskers") that make a "shhh" sound.
- After 2 weeks:
  - The people who wore earplugs could tolerate *less* sound than before.
  - The people who wore sound generators could tolerate *more* sound than before.
- This study showed that:
  - Adding sound makes it easier to tolerate sound.
  - Staying in quiet makes it harder to tolerate sound.

Bottom line

If everyday sounds bother you:

- Surrounding yourself with comfortable sound will help.
- Avoiding sound will make the problem worse.

How long does it take?

It can take weeks or months for your ears to adjust.

Talk to your audiologist if you have any questions.

[1]"Adaptive Calibration of Chronic Auditory Gain: Interim Findings," by C. Formby, L. P. Sherlock, & S. L. Gold, 2002, In *Proceedings of the VIIth International Tinnitus Seminar* (pp. 165–169) by R. Patuzzi (Ed.), Crawley, Australia: University of Western Australia.

APPENDIX F

PTM

Progressive Tinnitus Management

Tinnitus Handicap Inventory

Instructions: The purpose of this questionnaire is to identify problems your tinnitus may be causing you. Check **Yes, Sometimes**, or **No** for each question. Do not skip a question.

		Yes (4)	*Sometimes (2)*	*No (0)*
1F	Because of your tinnitus, is it difficult for you to concentrate?	☐	☐	☐
2F	Does the loudness of your tinnitus make it difficult for you to hear people?	☐	☐	☐
3E	Does your tinnitus make you angry?	☐	☐	☐
4F	Does your tinnitus make you feel confused?	☐	☐	☐
5C	Because of your tinnitus, do you feel desperate?	☐	☐	☐
6E	Do you complain a great deal about your tinnitus?	☐	☐	☐
7F	Because of your tinnitus, do you have trouble falling to sleep at night?	☐	☐	☐
8C	Do you feel as though you cannot escape your tinnitus?	☐	☐	☐
9F	Does your tinnitus interfere with your ability to enjoy social activities (such as going out to dinner, to the movies)?	☐	☐	☐
10E	Because of your tinnitus, do you feel frustrated?	☐	☐	☐
11C	Because of your tinnitus, do you feel that you have a terrible disease?	☐	☐	☐
12F	Does your tinnitus make it difficult for you to enjoy life?	☐	☐	☐
13F	Does your tinnitus interfere with your job or household responsibilities?	☐	☐	☐
14F	Because of your tinnitus, do you find that you are often irritable?	☐	☐	☐
15F	Because of your tinnitus, is it difficult for you to read?	☐	☐	☐
16E	Does your tinnitus make you upset?	☐	☐	☐
17E	Do you feel that your tinnitus problem has placed stress on your relationship with members of your family and friends?	☐	☐	☐
18F	Do you find it difficult to focus your attention away from your tinnitus and on other things?	☐	☐	☐
19C	Do you feel that you have no control over your tinnitus?	☐	☐	☐
20F	Because of your tinnitus, do you often feel tired?	☐	☐	☐
21E	Because of your tinnitus, do you feel depressed?	☐	☐	☐
22E	Does your tinnitus make you feel anxious?	☐	☐	☐
23C	Do you feel that you can no longer cope with your tinnitus?	☐	☐	☐

continues

Appendix F continued

		Yes (4)	Sometimes (2)	No (0)
24F	Does your tinnitus get worse when you are under stress?	☐	☐	☐
25E	Does your tinnitus make you feel insecure?	☐	☐	☐
	Total	____	____	____

F denotes an item on the functional subscale; E, an item on the emotional subscale; and C, an item on the catastrophic response subscale.

From "Development of the Tinnitus Handicap Inventory," by C. W. Newman, G. P. Jacobson, & J. B. Spitzer, 1996, *Archives of Otolaryngology-Head and Neck Surgery, 122,* 143–148. Reprinted with permission.

TINNITUS HANDICAP INVENTORY
Screening Version

Instructions: The purpose of this questionnaire is to identify problems your tinnitus may be causing you. Check **Yes**, **Sometimes**, or **No** for each question. Do not skip a question.

		Yes (4)	*Sometimes (2)*	*No (0)*
1	Because of your tinnitus, is it difficult for you to concentrate?	☐	☐	☐
2	Do you complain a great deal regarding your tinnitus?	☐	☐	☐
3	Do you feel as though you cannot escape your tinnitus?	☐	☐	☐
4	Does your tinnitus make you feel confused?	☐	☐	☐
5	Because of your tinnitus, do you feel frustrated?	☐	☐	☐
6	Do you feel that you can no longer cope with your tinnitus?	☐	☐	☐
7	Does your tinnitus make it difficult for you to enjoy life?	☐	☐	☐
8	Does your tinnitus make you upset?	☐	☐	☐
9	Because of your tinnitus, do you have trouble falling asleep at night?	☐	☐	☐
10	Because of your tinnitus, do you feel depressed?	☐	☐	☐
	Total	____	____	____

From "Development and Psychometric Adequacy of the Screening Version of the Tinnitus Handicap Inventory," by C. W. Newman, S. A. Sandridge, & L. Bolek, 2008, *Otology and Neurotology, 29*(3), 276–281. Reprinted with permission.

APPENDIX G

PTM

Progressive Tinnitus Management

Hearing Handicap Inventory—E
Screening Version

Please answer the following questions based on your last two weeks.

		Yes (4)	*Sometimes (2)*	*No (0)*
1.	Does a hearing problem cause you to feel embarrassed when you meet new people?	☐	☐	☐
2.	Does a hearing problem cause you to feel frustrated when talking to members of your family?	☐	☐	☐
3.	Do you have difficulty when someone speaks in a whisper?	☐	☐	☐
4.	Do you feel handicapped by a hearing problem?	☐	☐	☐
5.	Does a hearing problem cause you difficulty when visiting friends, relatives, or neighbors?	☐	☐	☐
6.	Does a hearing problem cause you to attend religious services less often than you would like?	☐	☐	☐
7.	Does a hearing problem cause you to have arguments with family members?	☐	☐	☐
8.	Does a hearing problem cause you difficulty when listening to TV or radio?	☐	☐	☐
9.	Do you feel that any difficulty with your hearing limits or hampers your personal or social life?	☐	☐	☐
10.	Does a hearing problem cause you difficulty when in a restaurant with relatives or friends?	☐	☐	☐
	Total	____	____	____

From "Identification of Elderly People with Hearing Problems," by I. M. Ventry, & B. E. Weinstein, 1983, *Asha, 25(7)*, 37–42. Reprinted with permission.

APPENDIX H

PTM

Progressive Tinnitus Management

Tinnitus Problem Checklist

1. My **most** bothersome tinnitus situation is:

- ☐ Falling asleep at night
- ☐ Staying asleep at night
- ☐ Waking up in the morning
- ☐ Reading
- ☐ Working at the computer
- ☐ Relaxing in my recliner
- ☐ Napping during the day
- ☐ Planning activities
- ☐ Driving
- ☐ Other ____________________

Write your answer on #1 of the Sound Plan Worksheet. Copies of the worksheet can be found at the end of the self-help workbook.[1]

2. My **second most** bothersome tinnitus situation is:

- ☐ Falling asleep at night
- ☐ Staying asleep at night
- ☐ Waking up in the morning
- ☐ Reading
- ☐ Working at the computer
- ☐ Relaxing in my recliner
- ☐ Napping during the day
- ☐ Planning activities
- ☐ Driving
- ☐ Other ____________________

Write your answer on #1 of a *separate* Sound Plan Worksheet.

3. My **third most** bothersome tinnitus situation is:

- ☐ Falling asleep at night
- ☐ Staying asleep at night
- ☐ Waking up in the morning
- ☐ Reading
- ☐ Working at the computer
- ☐ Relaxing in my recliner
- ☐ Napping during the day
- ☐ Planning activities
- ☐ Driving
- ☐ Other ____________________

Write your answer on #1 of a *separate* Sound Plan Worksheet.

[1] *How to Manage Your Tinnitus: A Step-by-Step Workbook*, by J. A. Henry, T. L. Zaugg, P. M. Myers, & C. M. Kendall, 2010, San Diego, CA: Plural Publishing, Inc. Reprinted with permission.

APPENDIX I

PTM
Progressive Tinnitus Management

Flowchart for Assessment and Fitting of Ear-Level Instruments

Level 1 is the triage level and does not involve audiology services. The focus of this flowchart is to show how decisions normally are made regarding the evaluation and fitting of different ear-level instruments (hearing aids, noise generators, and combination instruments) that can be used for tinnitus management. As noted in Chapter 5, new models of combination instruments do not sacrifice hearing aid performance. These devices can be fitted at Level 2, but it is recommended that the sound/noise generator be turned off until after the patient has attended at least the first session of Level 3 Group Education.

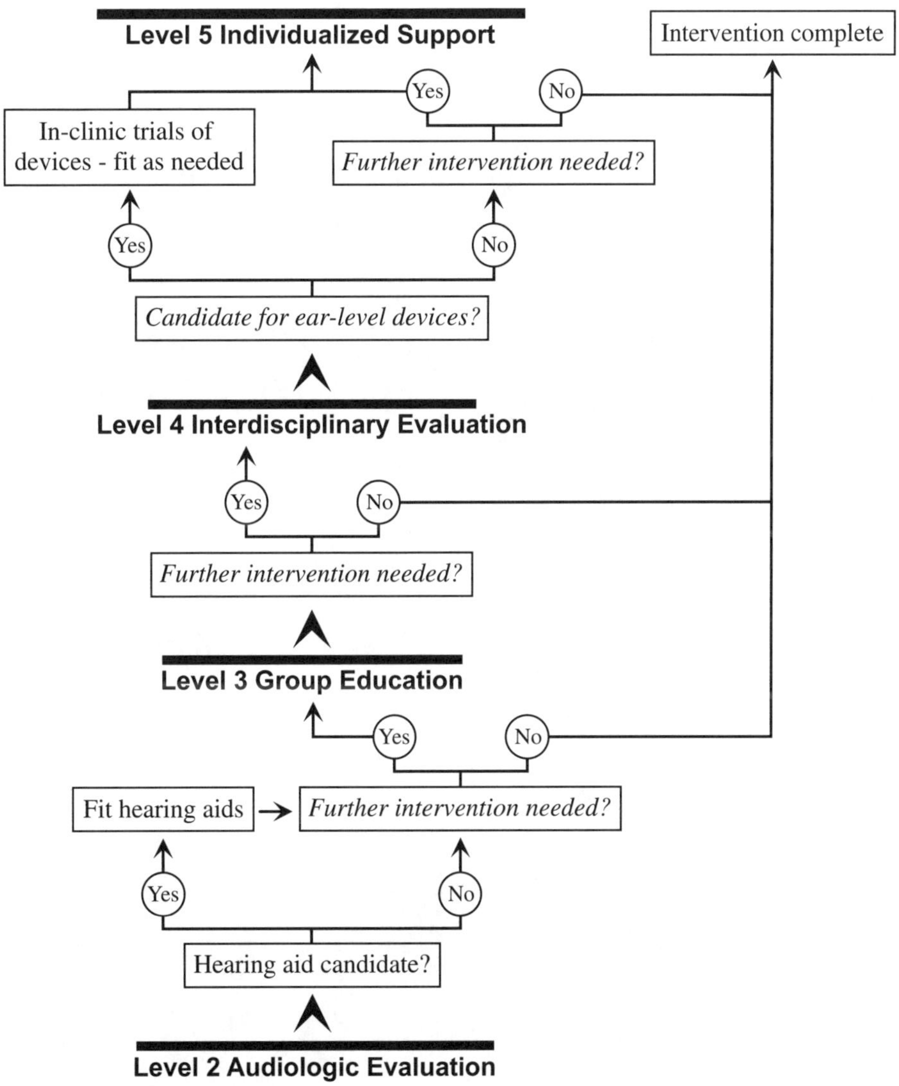

APPENDIX

J

PTM

Progressive Tinnitus Management

Level 2 Audiologic Evaluation: Special Considerations for Hearing Aids

1. **Some patients are obvious hearing aid candidates. Fit them with hearing aids as you normally would, except try to incorporate the following hearing aid features that are important for tinnitus management:**

   A. Use open-ear fitting if possible (or maximum venting)
   B. Use feedback reduction circuitry to enable most open fitting
   C. Ensure that any feature for reducing circuit noise (e.g., expansion) can be disabled—internal/floor noise can be desirable for tinnitus
   D. Ensure that any feature for reducing environmental noise can be disabled

2. **Some patients are borderline hearing aid candidates. Be more open to trying hearing aids with these patients than for patients who do not have a tinnitus problem. Explain to these patients that hearing aids can help with both hearing problems and tinnitus problems.**

   A. Consider hearing aids for borderline hearing aid candidates if:
      1) Patient is motivated to try hearing aids for the purpose of improving communicative and other hearing problems
         AND/OR
      2) Patient is motivated to try hearing aids for the purpose of amplifying environmental sound to reduce tinnitus intrusiveness

   B. Incorporate the hearing aid features listed above that are important for tinnitus management.

APPENDIX K

Sound Tolerance Interview

[Note to clinician: Use this interview only if the patient already has reported a sound tolerance problem.]

Instructions to patients: You told me that some sounds are too loud for you when they seem normal to other people around you. We refer to this as **trouble tolerating sound**. I am going to ask you some questions about trouble tolerating sound. When you answer the questions, think back to how you have been doing over the last week.

1. **Do you wear hearing aids?**

   ☐ No—go to Question 2
   ☐ Yes

   (If YES) Are everyday sounds too loud when you are wearing your hearing aids?

   ☐ No
   ☐ Yes

   (If YES) Are everyday sounds too loud when you are ***not*** wearing your hearing aids?

   ☐ No
   ☐ Yes

   [Note to clinician: If the sound tolerance problem appears to be caused by sounds amplified by hearing aids, consider making compression, MPO, and/or other adjustments to the aids to improve comfort. If the patient is not bothered by sound when unaided, then it is possible that all that is needed is to adjust the hearing aids for comfort.]

2. ***How* does trouble tolerating sound affect your life?**

   ____

3. **On a scale of 0 to 10, *how much* does trouble tolerating sound affect your life? ("0" would be "not at all"; "10" would be "as much as you can imagine.")**

   (not at all) 0 1 2 3 4 5 6 7 8 9 10 **(as much as you can imagine)**

4. **What kinds of sounds are too loud for you?**

   [Clinician: check all categories that apply; circle any sounds that the patient identifies as a problem; write in any additional sounds mentioned by the patient.]

   ☐ **Higher pitched sounds** (squeals, squeaks, beeps, whistles, rings, ______________)
   ☐ **Lower pitched sounds** (bass from radio, next-door music, ______________)

continues

Appendix K continued

- ☐ **Traffic (warning) sounds** (emergency vehicle sirens, car horns, backup beeper on truck/van, ______________________________)
- ☐ **Traffic (background) sounds** (road noise, road construction, diesel engines, garbage trucks, ______________________________)
- ☐ **Sudden impact sounds** (door slam, car backfiring, objects dropping on floor, dishes clattering, ______________________________)
- ☐ **Voices** (television, radio, movies, children's voices, dog barking, ______________________________)
- ☐ **Other** (describe ______________________________)

5. **I'm going to read a list of activities. I want you to tell me how often trouble tolerating sound is a problem during these activities.**

   [Clinician: check ***avoids*** if the patient avoids any of these activities due to trouble tolerating sound; if an activity is avoided, you *can* check two boxes for that activity.]

	Never	*Rarely*	*Sometimes*	*Often*	*Always*	*N/A*	**Avoids**
a. Concerts?	☐	☐	☐	☐	☐	☐	☐
b. Shopping?	☐	☐	☐	☐	☐	☐	☐
c. Movies?	☐	☐	☐	☐	☐	☐	☐
d. Work? (select N/A if retired)	☐	☐	☐	☐	☐	☐	☐
e. Day-to-day responsibilities outside of work?	☐	☐	☐	☐	☐	☐	☐
f. Going to restaurants?	☐	☐	☐	☐	☐	☐	☐
g. Driving?	☐	☐	☐	☐	☐	☐	☐
h. Participating in or observing sports events?	☐	☐	☐	☐	☐	☐	☐
i. Attending church?	☐	☐	☐	☐	☐	☐	☐
j. Housekeeping activities?	☐	☐	☐	☐	☐	☐	☐
k. Child care?	☐	☐	☐	☐	☐	☐	☐
l. Social activities?	☐	☐	☐	☐	☐	☐	☐
m. Anything else? ______________	☐	☐	☐	☐	☐	☐	☐

6. **Do you ever use earplugs or earmuffs?**
   - ☐ No → **Interview is complete**
   - ☐ Yes

(If YES) What percentage of your awake time do you use earplugs or earmuffs?

☐ 5%	☐ 30%	☐ 55%	☐ 80%
☐ 10%	☐ 35%	☐ 60%	☐ 85%
☐ 15%	☐ 40%	☐ 65%	☐ 90%
☐ 20%	☐ 45%	☐ 70%	☐ 95%
☐ 25%	☐ 50%	☐ 75%	☐ 100%

(If YES) Do you ever use earplugs or earmuffs in fairly quiet situations?

☐ No ☐ Yes

[Note to clinician: Some patients have difficulty understanding the point of this question. Another way to phrase it is: *"Do you ever use earplugs or earmuffs because sounds are too loud for you when they seem normal to other people around you?"* The concern is that people with sound tolerance problems may wear hearing protection in fairly quiet situations out of fear that they will encounter an uncomfortably loud sound. That behavior would be considered *overprotecting* ears, and is likely to cause the sound tolerance problem to worsen. These patients need to understand that use of hearing protection can lead to greater sensitivity to sound, thus exacerbating their sound tolerance problem.]

[Clinician: does patient overprotect ears due to problems with sound tolerance?]

☐ No ☐ Yes

Adapted with permission from: *Tinnitus Retraining Therapy: Clinical Guidelines*, by J. A. Henry, D. R. Trune, M. J. A. Robb, & P. J. Jastreboff, 2007, San Diego, CA: Plural Publishing, Inc.

APPENDIX

L

PTM

Progressive Tinnitus Management

Sound Tolerance Worksheet

Things I can do	1. When and where will I do this?	2. How will I do this?	3. Comments	4. Am I doing better?
Surround myself with comfortable sound				After 1 month:
Listen to sounds I enjoy				After 2 months:
Use earplugs or earmuffs only when needed				After 3 months:

APPENDIX

M

PTM

Progressive Tinnitus Management

Loudness Discomfort Levels— Clinical Guide

1. Definitions
   A. Hyperacusis: significantly reduced tolerance to sound that is restricted to auditory pathways
   B. Misophonia: dislike of sound due to emotional reactions caused by sound
   C. Phonophobia: specific case of misophonia when fear of sound is involved
   D. Loudness recruitment: abnormally rapid growth of loudness caused by loss of outer hair cells
   E. LDL: threshold level of physical (not emotional) discomfort for a sound
2. LDL testing
   A. General guidelines
      1. Patient must understand instructions to ensure proper response
      2. Test at octave frequencies between 1 and 8 kHz
      3. Test each ear separately
      4. Order testing from lowest to highest frequency
      5. Present tones for 1–2 seconds each
      6. Obtain LDLs twice within a session (test each ear, then repeat all testing)
      7. Record only the second set of LDLs
   B. Specific procedures
      1. Instruct: *"You will listen to different tones. Each tone will be made slightly louder in steps. Tell me when the loudness of the tone would be OK for 3 seconds, but would not be OK for more than 3 seconds."*
      2. Present 1-kHz tone at approximate MCL (50–60 dB HL)
      3. Raise level in 5-dB steps until patient signals that LDL has been reached
      4. Starting levels at remaining frequencies should be about 20 dB below previous frequency's LDL
      5. When each ear has been tested once:
         - Repeat instructions to patient
         - Obtain second set of measures
         - Record second set of measures

APPENDIX

N

PTM

Progressive Tinnitus Management

Sound Plan Worksheet

1. Write down one bothersome tinnitus situation ______________________________

2. **Check one or more** of the three ways to use sound to manage the situation	3. **Write down the sounds** that you will try	4. **Write down the devices** you will use	5. Use your sound plan **over the next week. How helpful** was each sound after using it for 1 week?	6. **Comments** When you find something that works well (or not so well) please comment. You do not need to wait 1 week to write your comments.
☐ **Soothing sound** 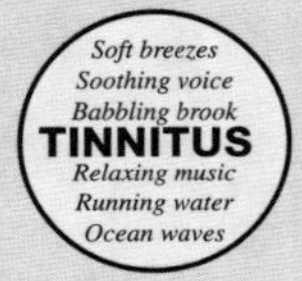	______ ______ ______	______ ______ ______	Not at all ☐ A little ☐ Moderately ☐ Very much ☐ Extremely ☐ ☐ ☐ ☐ ☐ ☐ ☐ ☐ ☐ ☐ ☐	______ ______ ______
☐ **Background sound** 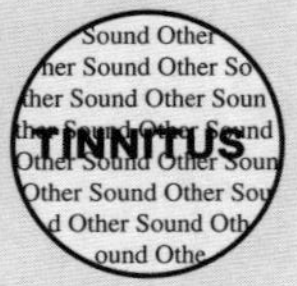	______ ______ ______	______ ______ ______	Not at all ☐ A little ☐ Moderately ☐ Very much ☐ Extremely ☐ ☐ ☐ ☐ ☐ ☐ ☐ ☐ ☐ ☐ ☐	______ ______ ______
☐ **Interesting sound** 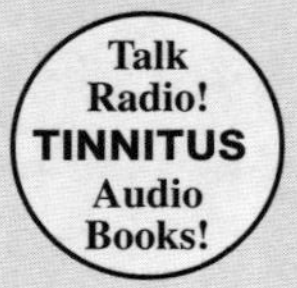	______ ______ ______	______ ______ ______	Not at all ☐ A little ☐ Moderately ☐ Very much ☐ Extremely ☐ ☐ ☐ ☐ ☐ ☐ ☐ ☐ ☐ ☐ ☐	______ ______ ______

APPENDIX

O

Relief Scale

Relief Scale

Instructions:

1. Choose a sound that you think will be soothing. A soothing sound will give you a sense of relief from stress or tension caused by tinnitus. (Tracks 9–14 on the CD in the back of the self-help workbook[1] have sounds that are soothing to many people.)
2. Adjust the volume of the sound until you find the level that is most soothing to you.
3. Answer the question "When I listen to this sound, how much relief from stress and tension do I feel?"

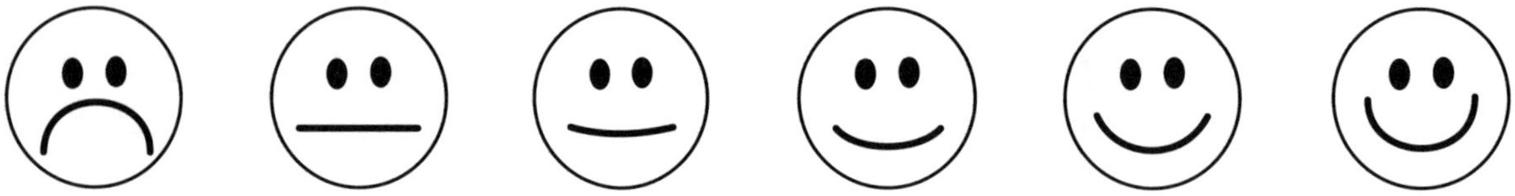

0	1	2	3	4	5
No relief	Slight relief	Mild relief	Moderate relief	Nearly complete relief	Complete relief

Write down the sound that you listened to	How much relief did the sound give you?					
	0	1	2	3	4	5
	0	1	2	3	4	5
	0	1	2	3	4	5
	0	1	2	3	4	5
	0	1	2	3	4	5
	0	1	2	3	4	5
	0	1	2	3	4	5
	0	1	2	3	4	5
	0	1	2	3	4	5
	0	1	2	3	4	5
	0	1	2	3	4	5
	0	1	2	3	4	5

[1] *How to Manage Your Tinnitus: A Step-by-Step Workbook,* by J. A. Henry, T. L. Zaugg, P. M. Myers, & C. M. Kendall, 2010, San Diego, CA: Plural Publishing, Inc. Reprinted with permission.

APPENDIX

P

Attention Scale

Attention Scale

Instructions:

1. Choose a sound that you think will keep your attention. (Tracks 15–19 on the CD in the back of the self-help workbook[1] have sounds that are interesting to many people.)
2. Listen to the sound for at least 1 minute.
3. Choose the percent of attention focused on the sound while listening to it.

Attention focused on:

Tinnitus **Other Sound**

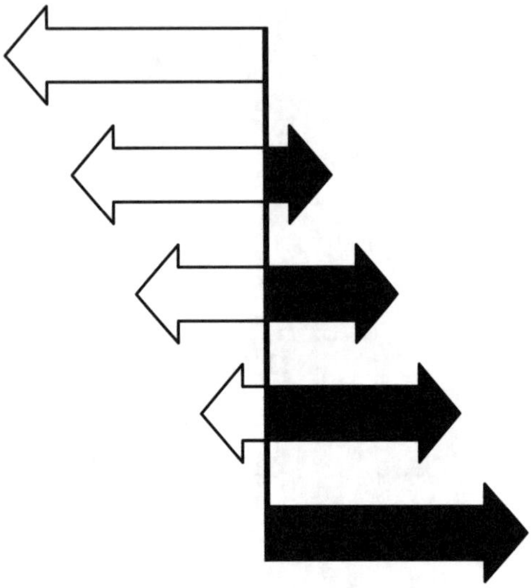

0% of attention focused on Other Sound

25% of attention focused on Other Sound

50% of attention focused on Other Sound

75% of attention focused on Other Sound

100% of attention focused on Other Sound

Write down the sound that you listened to	How much of your attention was focused on the "Other Sound"?				
	0%	25%	50%	75%	100%
	0%	25%	50%	75%	100%
	0%	25%	50%	75%	100%
	0%	25%	50%	75%	100%
	0%	25%	50%	75%	100%
	0%	25%	50%	75%	100%
	0%	25%	50%	75%	100%
	0%	25%	50%	75%	100%
	0%	25%	50%	75%	100%

[1]*How to Manage Your Tinnitus: A Step-by-Step Workbook,* by J. A. Henry, T. L. Zaugg, P. M. Myers, & C. M. Kendall, 2010, San Diego, CA: Plural Publishing, Inc. Reprinted with permission.

APPENDIX

Q

Tinnitus Contrast Activity

Tinnitus Contrast Activity

Tinnitus Contrast Activity

1. Spend a few moments listening to your tinnitus in quiet.
2. Now turn on some background sound. The sound should be pleasant or neutral. (Tracks 20–23 on the CD in the back of the self-help workbook[1] have sounds that are background sound to many people.)
3. Adjust the volume to a comfortable level.
4. Notice the reduced contrast.
5. Reducing contrast makes it easier to ignore your tinnitus.

TINNITUS	**ELEVATOR MUSIC** **RADIO STATIC** **CLASSICAL MUSIC** **ELECTRIC FAN** **WHITE NOISE GUITAR MUSIC** **TINNITUS** **TRAFFIC NOISE WIND NOISE** **AIR CONDITIONER** **NEW AGE MUSIC** **FOUNTAIN NOISE** **FISH TANK NOISE**

Write down the sound that you listened to	Write any comments you have about using this sound as background sound

[1]*How to Manage Your Tinnitus: A Step-by-Step Workbook*, by J. A. Henry, T. L. Zaugg, P. M. Myers, & C. M. Kendall, 2010, San Diego, CA: Plural Publishing, Inc. Reprinted with permission.

APPENDIX R

PTM

Progressive Tinnitus Management

Level 4 Interdisciplinary Evaluation: Tinnitus Interview

Clinicians: This interview is intended to be administered immediately after administering the Tinnitus and Hearing Survey and thoroughly discussing the results with the patient. (Please note that this interview does not cover tinnitus-specific information that most likely was covered during the case history performed during the Level 2 Audiologic Evaluation. It may be helpful to review the case history before administering this interview.)

1. Does the loudness of your tinnitus change *on its own*?

- ☐ No → Go to #2
- ☐ Yes → How often does it change?
  - ☐ Never
  - ☐ Several times per month
  - ☐ Several times per week
  - ☐ Several times per day
  - ☐ Several times per hour

2. Do sounds ever change the loudness of your tinnitus?

☐ No effect → Go to #3 ☐ Softer → Go to #3

☐ Louder

(if "LOUDER") What kinds of sounds make your tinnitus louder? [Clinician: check all categories that apply; circle any sounds that the patient identifies as a problem; write in any additional sounds mentioned by the patient.]

☐ Very loud sounds/activities that would be expected to make the tinnitus louder (firing a gun, attending a concert, using power tools, ____________________) [Clinician: If this is the only response from the patient, then exacerbation of tinnitus by sound would be considered a normal effect.]

☐ Higher pitched sounds (squeals, squeaks, beeps, whistles, rings, ____________________)

☐ Lower pitched sounds (bass from radio, ____________________)

☐ Traffic (warning) sounds (emergency vehicle sirens, car horns, backup beeper on truck/van, ____________________)

☐ Traffic (background) sounds (road noise, road construction, diesel engines, garbage trucks, ____________________)

☐ Sudden impact sounds (door slam, car backfiring, objects dropping on floor, dishes clattering, ____________________)

continues

Appendix R continued

☐ Voices (television, radio, movies, children's voices, dog barking, ____________________)

☐ Other (describe) ____

When sound makes your tinnitus louder, how long does the change last?

☐ 1–2 ☐ Second(s)
☐ 3–4 ☐ Minute(s)
☐ 5–10 ☐ Hour(s)
☐ more than 10 ☐ Day(s)

3. How does your tinnitus affect you (not including trouble hearing or understanding speech)?

____

____

4. Please tell me about everything you tried for your tinnitus prior to PTM. For each effort, what were you hoping would happen, and what actually did happen? [Clinician: Sometimes a pattern will emerge showing that the patient has made repeated (unsuccessful) attempts to make the tinnitus quieter, resulting in frustration and distress. If this is the case, try to ensure that the patient begins to see this pattern more clearly.]

What have you tried for tinnitus prior to PTM?	***What were you hoping would happen?***	***What actually did happen?***
______________	______________	______________
______________	______________	______________
______________	______________	______________
______________	______________	______________
______________	______________	______________
______________	______________	______________
______________	______________	______________

5. Please tell me about the sounds you have used to manage your reactions to tinnitus since starting PTM. For each sound you tried, what were you hoping would happen, and what actually did happen? [Clinician: if the patient has the Sound Plan Worksheets that were used during Level 3, these can be used to guide this interaction. It also is important to reinforce the idea that with PTM the goal is not to change the tinnitus, but rather to change how one feels.]

What sounds have you used to manage reactions to tinnitus during PTM?	***What were you hoping would happen?***	***What actually did happen?***
________________	________________	________________
________________	________________	________________
________________	________________	________________
________________	________________	________________
________________	________________	________________
________________	________________	________________
________________	________________	________________

continues

Appendix R continued

6. If we decide to move ahead with one-on-one support, then we will be making plans for using sound to manage your reactions to tinnitus. It will be helpful to have a list of sound producing devices that you have available to you. Which of the following devices do you own? [Clinician: For each type of device listed below that the patient owns, provide additional details. For instance, if patients report they own a radio, ask: how many radios, if any of them are portable, and if not portable, where it is located. For each device the patient owns, ask how it currently is being used relative to tinnitus management.]

Type of device	*How many are available?*	*Are any portable?*	*If not portable, where is it located?*	*How is it being used with respect to tinnitus?*
☐ Television				
☐ Radio				
☐ MP3 player				
☐ CD player				
☐ Satellite radio				
☐ Table top sound generator ("sound spa")				
☐ Table top water fountain				
☐ Fan/air conditioner/ etc.				
☐ Music channels on cable or satellite TV				
☐ Computer with internet access (to access radio stations, podcasts, and other sources of sound)				
☐ Cell phone capable of playing music				
☐ Other				

APPENDIX S

PTM

Progressive Tinnitus Management

Hospital Anxiety and Depression Scale (HADS)

Emotions play an important part in most illnesses. The more your health care providers know about your feelings the better they will be able to help you.

This questionnaire is designed to help your health care providers know how you feel. Read each item and put a checkmark in the box next to the reply that best describes how you have been feeling in the past week. Ignore the numbers printed on the left side.

Don't take too long thinking over your replies. Your first reaction to each item will probably be the most accurate response.

A **I feel tense or "wound up":**
3 ☐ Most of the time
2 ☐ A lot of the time
1 ☐ From time to time, occasionally
0 ☐ Not at all

D **I still enjoy the things I used to enjoy:**
0 ☐ Definitely as much
1 ☐ Not quite so much
2 ☐ Only a little
3 ☐ Hardly at all

A **I get a sort of frightened feeling as if something awful is about to happen:**
3 ☐ Very definitely and quite badly
2 ☐ Yes, but not too badly
1 ☐ A little, but it doesn't worry me
0 ☐ Not at all

D **I can laugh and see the funny side of things:**
0 ☐ As much as I always could
1 ☐ Not quite so much now
2 ☐ Definitely not so much now
3 ☐ Not at all

A **Worrying thoughts go through my mind:**
3 ☐ A great deal of the time
2 ☐ A lot of the time
1 ☐ From time to time, but not too often
0 ☐ Only occasionally

D **I feel cheerful:**
3 ☐ Not at all
2 ☐ Not often
1 ☐ Sometimes
0 ☐ Most of the time

A **I can sit at ease and feel relaxed:**
0 ☐ Definitely
1 ☐ Usually
2 ☐ Not often
3 ☐ Not at all

D **I feel as if I am slowed down:**
3 ☐ Nearly all the time
2 ☐ Very often
1 ☐ Sometimes
0 ☐ Not at all

A **I get a sort of frightened feeling like "butterflies" in the stomach:**
0 ☐ Not at all
1 ☐ Occasionally
2 ☐ Quite often
3 ☐ Very often

D **I have lost interest in my appearance:**
3 ☐ Definitely
2 ☐ I don't take as much care as I should
1 ☐ I may not take quite as much care
0 ☐ I take just as much care as ever

continues

Appendix S continued

A **I feel restless as if I have to be on the move:**

3 ☐ Very much indeed
2 ☐ Quite a lot
1 ☐ Not very much
0 ☐ Not at all

D **I look forward with enjoyment to things:**

0 ☐ As much as I ever did
1 ☐ Rather less than I used to
2 ☐ Definitely less than I used to
3 ☐ Hardly at all

A **I get sudden feelings of panic:**

3 ☐ Very often indeed
2 ☐ Quite often
1 ☐ Not very often
0 ☐ Not at all

D **I can enjoy a good book or radio or TV program:**

0 ☐ Often
1 ☐ Sometimes
2 ☐ Not often
3 ☐ Very seldom

Totals	Clinician: add the individual scores for the "A's" (anxiety), and then for the "D's" (depression). This is a screening tool only, it is not diagnostic. 0–7 normal 8–10 referral for further evaluation may be helpful 11–21 referral for further evaluation likely to be helpful

From "The Hospital Anxiety and Depression Scale," by A. S. Zigmond, & R. P. Snaith, 1983, *Acta Psychiatrica Scandinavica, 67*(6), 361–370. Reprinted with permission.

APPENDIX T

PTM

Progressive Tinnitus Management

The Primary Care PTSD Screen (PC-PTSD)

Description

The PC-PTSD is a four-item screen that was designed for use in primary care and other medical settings and currently is used to screen for PTSD in veterans at the VA. The screen includes an introductory sentence to cue respondents to traumatic events. The authors suggest that in most circumstances the results of the PC-PTSD should be considered "positive" if a patient answers "yes" to any three items. A cutoff score of 2 can be used to optimize sensitivity. Those screening positive should then be assessed with a structured interview for PTSD. The screen does not include a list of potentially traumatic events.

Scale

Instructions

In your life, have you ever had any experience that was so frightening, horrible, or upsetting that, in the past month, you:

1. Have had nightmares about it or thought about it when you did not want to? **YES / NO**
2. Tried hard not to think about it or went out of your way to avoid situations that reminded you of it? **YES / NO**
3. Were constantly on guard, watchful, or easily startled? **YES / NO**
4. Felt numb or detached from others, activities, or your surroundings? **YES / NO**

Current research suggests that the results of the PC-PTSD should be considered "positive" if a patient answers "yes" to any three items.

References

Prins, A., Ouimette, P., Kimerling, R., Cameron, R. P., Hugelshofer, D. S., Shaw-Hegwer, J., . . . Sheikh, J. I. (2003). The primary care PTSD screen (PC–PTSD): Development and operating characteristics. *Primary Care Psychiatry, 9*, 9–14

Prins, A., Ouimette, P., Kimerling, R., Cameron, R. P., Hugelshofer, D. S., Shaw-Hegwer, J., . . . Sheikh, J. I. (2004). The primary care PTSD screen (PC–PTSD): Corrigendum. *Primary Care Psychiatry, 9*, 151

Additional Reviews

Orsillo, S. M. (2001). Measures for acute stress disorder and posttraumatic stress disorder. In M. M. Antony & S. M. Orsillo (Eds.), *Practitioner's guide to empirically based measures of anxiety* (pp. 255–307). New York, NY: KluwerAcademic/Plenum. PILOTS ID 24368 (p. 299).

Norris, F. H., & Hamblen, J. L. (2004). Standardized self-report measures of civilian trauma and PTSD. In J. P. Wilson, T. M. Keane & T. Martin (Eds.), *Assessing psychological trauma and PTSD* (pp. 63–102). New York, NY: Guilford Press. PILOTS ID 18638 (p. 71).

APPENDIX

U

PTM

Progressive Tinnitus Management

Epworth Sleepiness Scale

The Epworth Sleepiness Scale is used to determine the level of daytime sleepiness. A score of 10 or more is considered sleepy. A score of 18 or more is very sleepy. If you score 10 or more on this test, you should consider whether you are obtaining adequate sleep, need to improve your sleep hygiene and/or need to see a sleep specialist. These issues should be discussed with your personal physician.

Use the following scale to choose the most appropriate number for each situation:

0 = would *never* doze or sleep.
1 = *slight* chance of dozing or sleeping
2 = *moderate* chance of dozing or sleeping
3 = *high* chance of dozing or sleeping

Fill in your answers and see where you stand.

Situation	*Chance of Dozing or Sleeping*
1. Sitting and reading	_____
2. Watching TV	_____
3. Sitting inactive in a public place	_____
4. Being a passenger in a motor vehicle for an hour or more	_____
5. Lying down in the afternoon	_____
6. Sitting and talking to someone	_____
7. Sitting quietly after lunch (no alcohol)	_____
8. Stopped for a few minutes in traffic while driving	_____
Total score (add the scores up) (This is your Epworth score)	_____

APPENDIX V

PTM

Progressive Tinnitus Management

Level 4 Interdisciplinary Evaluation: Guide to Trial Use of Ear-Level Instruments

1. If your patient is an *obvious hearing aid candidate* follow the procedures outlined in the following forms (any order is acceptable):
   1. In-Clinic Trial Use of Hearing Aids (Appendix W) AND
   2. In-Clinic Trial Use of Combination Instruments (Appendix X)
      Note: Whether or not the patient is currently wearing hearing aids, follow the procedures outlined in both forms.

2. If your patient is a *borderline hearing aid candidate* follow the procedures outlined in the following forms (any order is acceptable):
   1. In-Clinic Trial Use of Hearing Aids (Appendix W) AND
   2. In-Clinic Trial Use of Combination Instruments (Appendix X) AND
   3. In-Clinic Trial Use of Noise Generators (Appendix Y)
      Note: Whether or not the patient is currently wearing hearing aids, follow the procedures outlined in all three forms.

3. If your patient is *not a hearing aid candidate* follow the procedures outlined in the following form:
   1. In-Clinic Trial Use of Noise Generators (Appendix Y)

After trying all instruments, discuss the following points:

- [Clinician: Ear-level instruments can improve hearing (which makes Interesting Sound more accessible), give a sense of relief, and provide a convenient source of Background Sound. Any or all of these effects are useful for managing tinnitus. The patient must be aware of these effects and choose which effect(s) is most important to him/her in making the final decision. Use the following discussion points and questions to make a decision about which, if any, instruments will be used during Level 5. Have the patient's completed Sound Plan Worksheet(s) available to look at during this discussion.]
- Any instruments you use should not be annoying at all
- Ear-level instruments can provide Soothing Sound (but even if they don't they still can be useful for managing tinnitus)
  - Did any of the instruments give you a sense of relief from tinnitus?
    - If yes, which instruments gave you the best sense of relief?
- *Remember, any ear-level device can provide a convenient source of Background Sound throughout the day—this alone can be helpful to manage tinnitus*
- (If hearing aids or combination instruments were tried) Improving hearing can make it easier to use Interesting Sound to manage tinnitus
  - Which instruments gave you the best hearing ability?
  - Do you think any of the instruments you tried today would make it easier for you to use Interesting Sound to manage tinnitus?
- Do you think any of the instruments you tried today could be helpful?
  - Which instruments would you most likely use?

APPENDIX W

PTM
Progressive Tinnitus Management

Level 4 Interdisciplinary Evaluation: In-Clinic Trial Use of Hearing Aids

- Use one form for each type of hearing aid that is evaluated
- If the patient is already using hearing aids, perform the trial with his/her current hearing aids
- **Goal:** establish realistic, experience-based judgment about the effectiveness of hearing aids for managing both hearing and tinnitus problems
- For each trial, escort patient through different acoustic environments
  a) *Quiet* environment (e.g., waiting area—not a sound booth)
  b) *Mildly noisy* environment (e.g., hallway)
  c) *Noisy* environment (e.g., dining area)

Conducting the Trial

☐ Adjust hearing aids to target gain using real-ear (adjust for comfort as needed)

	Acoustic environment			
Ask these questions:	***Quiet***	***Mildly noisy***	***Noisy***	***Comments***
Does the sound from the device(s) bother you? [Clinician: if "yes" try to adjust instruments to eliminate annoyance.]	Yes No	Yes No	Yes No	
With these instruments, is your hearing the same, better, or worse than without the instruments?	Same Better Worse	Same Better Worse	Same Better Worse	
With these instruments, how much relief do you feel from your tinnitus? [Clinician: Use the Relief Scale below.]	0 1 2 3 4 5	0 1 2 3 4 5	0 1 2 3 4 5	

Relief Scale

0	1	2	3	4	5
No relief	Slight relief	Mild relief	Moderate relief	Nearly complete relief	Complete relief

APPENDIX X

PTM

Progressive Tinnitus Management

Level 4 Interdisciplinary Evaluation: In-Clinic Trial Use of Combination Instruments

- Use one form for each type of combination instrument that is evaluated
- **Goal:** establish realistic, experience-based judgment about the effectiveness of combination instruments for managing both hearing and tinnitus problems
- For each trial, escort patient through different acoustic environments
  a) *Quiet* environment (e.g., waiting area—not a sound booth)
  b) *Mildly noisy* environment (e.g., hallway)
  c) *Noisy* environment (e.g., dining area)

Conducting the Trial

- ☐ First, adjust amplification portion of the combination instruments to target gain using real-ear equipment (adjust for comfort as needed)
- ☐ Second, adjust volume and frequency output of noise generator portion of the combination instruments to attempt to maximize sense of relief from tinnitus

	Acoustic environment			
Ask these questions:	***Quiet***	***Mildly noisy***	***Noisy***	***Comments***
Does the sound from the device(s) bother you? [Clinician: if "yes" try to adjust instruments to eliminate annoyance.]	Yes No	Yes No	Yes No	
With these instruments, is your hearing the same, better, or worse than without the instruments?	Same Better Worse	Same Better Worse	Same Better Worse	
With these instruments, how much relief do you feel from your tinnitus? [Clinician: Use the Relief Scale below.]	0 1 2 3 4 5	0 1 2 3 4 5	0 1 2 3 4 5	

Relief Scale

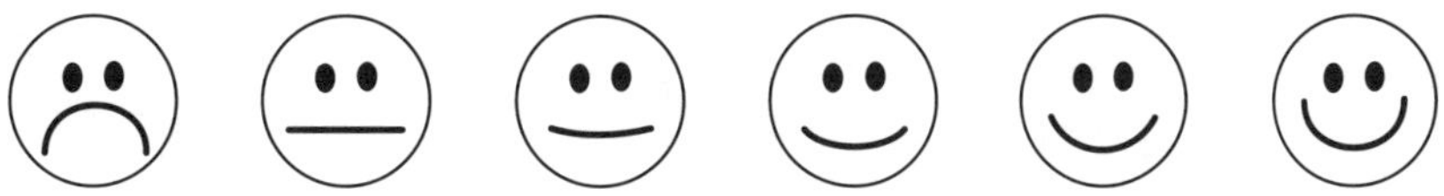

0	1	2	3	4	5
No relief	Slight relief	Mild relief	Moderate relief	Nearly complete relief	Complete relief

APPENDIX Y

PTM
Progressive Tinnitus Management

Level 4 Interdisciplinary Evaluation: In-Clinic Trial Use of Noise Generators

- Use one form for each type of noise/sound generator that is evaluated
- If the patient is already using hearing aids, have the patient complete the activity *In-Clinic Trial Use of Hearing Aids* (Appendix W) to reflect performance with their current hearing aids.
- **Goal:** establish realistic, experience-based judgment about the effectiveness of sound generators for managing tinnitus problems
- For each trial, escort patient through different acoustic environments
  a) *Quiet* environment (e.g., waiting area—not a sound booth)
  b) *Mildly noisy* environment (e.g., hallway)
  c) *Noisy* environment (e.g., dining area)

Conducting the Trial

☐ Adjust volume and frequency output of noise generator to attempt to maximize sense of relief from tinnitus.

	Acoustic environment			
Ask these questions:	***Quiet***	***Mildly noisy***	***Noisy***	***Comments***
Does the sound from the device(s) bother you? [Clinician: if "yes" try to adjust instruments to eliminate annoyance.]	Yes No	Yes No	Yes No	
With these instruments, is your hearing the same, better, or worse than without the instruments?	Same Better Worse	Same Better Worse	Same Better Worse	
With these instruments, how much relief do you feel from your tinnitus? [Clinician: Use the Relief Scale below.]	0 1 2 3 4 5	0 1 2 3 4 5	0 1 2 3 4 5	

Relief Scale

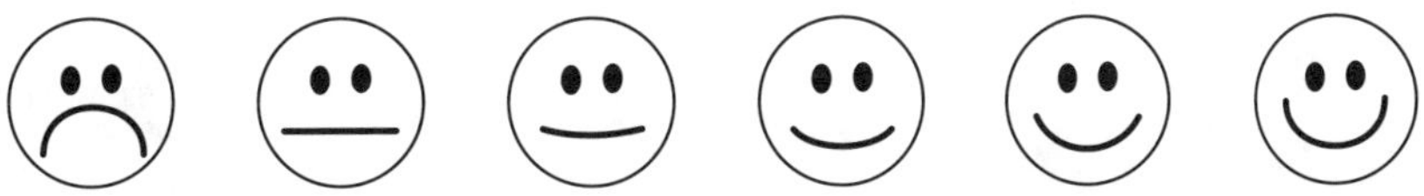

0	1	2	3	4	5
No relief	Slight relief	Mild relief	Moderate relief	Nearly complete relief	Complete relief

Descriptions of DVD and CD

A DVD and a CD are attached to the back cover of this handbook. The DVD contains four interactive videos. The first two videos model the education that is provided to patients during the two sessions of PTM Level 3 Group Education that are conducted by an audiologist. These two videos can be used to accomplish two purposes: (1) All clinicians who plan to lead Level 3 Group Education should first watch the videos while assuming the role of the patient—this will facilitate learning how to teach the Level 3 sessions. (2) The videos can be shown to groups of patients during the Level 3 Group Education instead of using the PowerPoint presentations that are provided in the attached CD. The third and fourth videos on the DVD provide demonstrations of two relaxation techniques—deep breathing and imagery. These relaxation videos can be used to supplement the Level 3 Group Education.

The CD contains PowerPoint files that should be used for the Level 3 Group Education sessions when conducting live presentations.

"Managing Your Tinnitus" DVD

Video 1: "Managing Your Tinnitus" for group viewing, Session 1

Length: 35:08

This is the first in a series of two video programs designed to be watched by a group of people. The two videos feature an interactive discussion of techniques for managing reactions to tinnitus. Researchers James Henry, Ph.D. and Tara Zaugg, Au.D. guide the viewers in developing a customized "sound plan" to manage reactions to tinnitus. This first video corresponds with the first session of Level 3 Group Education (see Chapter 7).

Video 2: "Managing Your Tinnitus" for group viewing, Session 2

Length: 27:00

This is the second in a series of two video programs designed to be watched by a group of people, and features an interactive discussion of techniques to use for tinnitus management. Researchers James Henry, Ph.D. and Tara Zaugg, Au.D. begin by reviewing important points from the first video session, then discuss ideas for choosing listening devices. This is followed by ideas for updating the viewers' sound plans, and a comparison of the different sound-based methods of tinnitus management. Finally, the researchers discuss other things viewers can do to manage their tinnitus.

Video 3: "Managing Your Tinnitus," Imagery Exercise

Length: 10:19

Tinnitus can cause stress and tension that prevents clear thinking and optimum functioning. This brief video guides the viewer through a powerful relaxation technique known as "Imagery." This exercise can be used any time to help the viewers get their mind off their tinnitus and help them feel calm and relaxed.

Video 4: "Managing Your Tinnitus," Deep Breathing Exercise

Length: 12:48

Tinnitus can cause stress and tension. Many people want their tinnitus to go away, or at least to be quieted. Unfortunately, there is no safe and consistent way to quiet tinnitus, but there are many ways to feel better by using techniques to relieve stress and tension. One of these techniques is called "Deep Breathing," and this video provides a relaxing, guided exercise to help the viewer learn the techniques to help them get their mind off their tinnitus so they can function more effectively.

CD with PowerPoint Files: "Managing Your Tinnitus: What to Do and How to Do It"— Sessions 1 and 2

The CD contains two PowerPoint files, three sound files, and a folder that contains Operations Files to make the programs work properly. The two PowerPoint files contain presentations titled *Managing Your Tinnitus: What to Do and How to Do It*—Sessions 1 and 2. The three sound files are linked to the Session 1 PowerPoint file.

These presentations were created to guide PTM Level 3 Group Education. Audiologists normally give the presentations, although they can be given by anyone who is proficient in the PTM education. Further information can be found in Chapter 7.

Index

L

M

N

O

P

Q

R

S

T

V

W